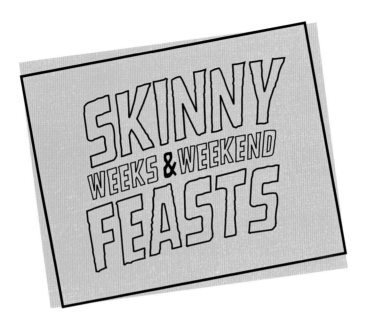

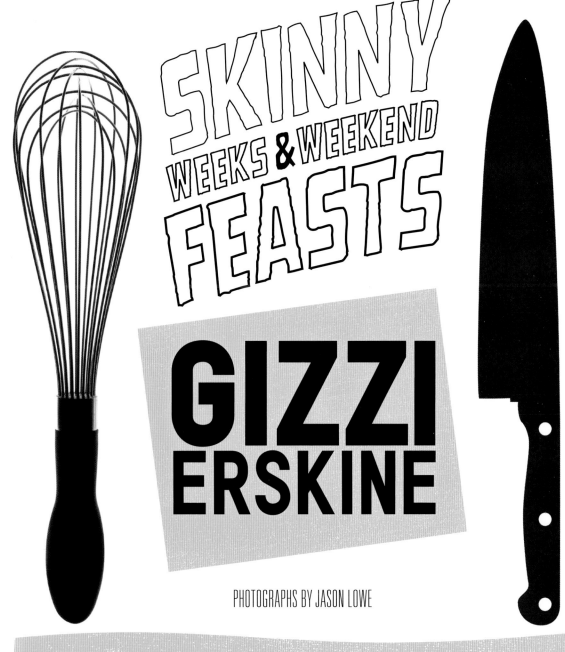

SKINNY
WEEKS & WEEKEND
FEASTS

GIZZI
ERSKINE

PHOTOGRAPHS BY JASON LOWE

XXX RATED for EXCITING, EXHILARATING, EXTRAORDINARY recipes • A REVELATORY BOOK OF TWO HALVES!! • BE AMAZED AT WHAT YOU CAN EAT!!

Quadrille
PUBLISHING

Publishing director: Jane O'Shea
Creative director: Helen Lewis
Project editor: Simon Davis
Design: Two Associates
Photographer: Jason Lowe
Illustrator: Dean Martin
Food stylist: Louisa Carter
Props stylist: Cynthia Inions
Production: James Finan

First published in 2013 by
Quadrille Publishing Limited
Alhambra House, 27-31
Charing Cross Road,
London WC2H 0LS
www.quadrille.co.uk

Reprinted in 2013
10 9 8 7 6 5 4 3 2

Text © 2013 Gizzi Erskine
Photography © 2013 Jason Lowe except pages 12–13, 102-3, 192
Illustration © 2013 Dean Martin
Design and layout © 2013 QuadrillePublishing Limited

Picture acknowledgments
Pages 12–13, 102-3, 192 © 2013 John Wright

978 184949 261 4

Printed in Italy

CONTENTS

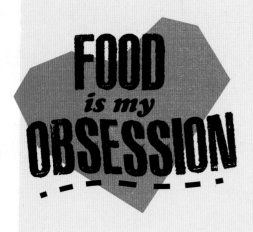

FOOD
is my
OBSESSION

I need to eat good food regularly or else I'm not the same person. And, like so many of us, every so often, I get carried away and eat too much. I find it hard to control what goes into my mouth because frankly, I want it all. My own personal vices are not actually that bad; it's portion control or that infamous 'inner-stop' button that I seem to lack.

As a result, I have the ability to put on weight – like a lot of girls, my weight goes up or down by a stone every 18 months. I've long been on the search for a way to nip this in the bud. And it's not like I don't have the answers on how to lose weight; I do!

When I presented *Cook Yourself Thin* my eyes were opened to the world of dieting in all its many varied shapes and forms. Yet the funny thing was, though people's diets and relationships with food were always very different, the thing that undid everyone's best intentions was always the same: denial. I saw that those people who didn't give themselves a bit of what they fancied occasionally were far more likely to quit their diet or get back into unhealthy routines once they had lost the weight. Interestingly, latest findings also indicate that those dieters who give themselves a day off a week will lose weight faster than those who diet strictly every day until they reach their target goal. Not only this BUT they will also maintain their weight better, as they will have introduced a healthy and feasible way of eating into their routine.

This idea bred this book. NOT entirely a diet book, but a book for FOOD LOVERS like me who want to get their weight and the way they eat UNDER CONTROL.

1500
CALORIES
PER DAY
ALLOWANCE

So how does it work? Essentially it is a book of two halves. The first, *Skinny Weeks*, is a guide to what you should eat for six days a week. During these days you will be looking at eating three meals and a couple of healthy snacks in between – aiming for a calorie intake of 1500 calories per day. A big mistake that many dieters make when they start a diet is to assume they can save calories by skipping meals, but it's actually much easier (and healthier) to stick to a diet if you spread your calories throughout the day. With this in mind you should aim for around 300 calories at breakfast, 400 calories for lunch and 600 calories for your evening meal – leaving you 200 calories for snacks (or even the occasional pud).

All of the recipes in the *Skinny Weeks* part of this book are designed to fit in with these calorie allowances – so all you need to do is choose a breakfast, a lunch, an evening meal and a couple of snacks. The fact is, the more you enjoy the food you're eating on your diet, the more you are likely to stick to it.

> **So I've filled this book with the sort of stuff you WANT to eat, weeding out the typical diet rabbit food and scouring the globe for DELICIOUS, SATISFYING food that just happens to be naturally HEALTHY.**

Now, here's the exciting bit: *Weekend Feasts* – one day a week you get to let your hair down, forget all about calories and choose one of the feasting options from the second part of book. I can make no claims that the recipes here are particularly 'healthy' (indeed, some are naughtier than others; check out the wickedness rating and make a decision on just how indulgent you want to be!) but they are all absolutely *irresistible*. Relax, unwind, cook up a storm and enjoy it, knowing that you've earned it. The *Skinny Weeks & Weekend Feasts* way of eating works best when giving yourself a day off at the weekend, but sometimes you might want to have this time off during the week instead. That's fine, too. And what's the end result? Well, following this plan you should lose between 1–2lb (1/2–1kg) a week. This may not sound like a lot, but after a couple of months that's over half a stone. And more than that, it's weight loss that is steady, pain-free and above all, achievable.

SO WHAT ARE YOU WAITING FOR?

It's time to throw out those faddy diet books and start to enjoy living life the *Skinny Weeks & Weekend Feasts* way...

Eating THE SKINNY WEEKS & WEEKEND FEASTS way

Skinny Weeks and Weekend Feasts is the antidote to drastic dietary changes, strict regimes or denial. It is, however based upon a few important principles, which are outlined below. Remember, our eating habits don't need revolutionising, they just need a bit of tweaking.

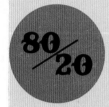

THE 80/20 RULE

Many nutritionists talk about the (80/20) rule – which is basically the concept that as long as you are virtuous and mindful about what you eat for 80% of the time, then what you do for the other 20% doesn't really matter. *The Skinny Weeks and Weekend Feasts* way of eating is underlined by this 80/20 ethos, while the recipes in the first half of this book also follow these additional principles:

Serve 20% less. We're bred to think we are only satisfied by a full plate. By taking a fifth off your plate you will reduce your calorie intake by 20% without even trying. Your stomach doesn't need to be at full capacity – in fact, it's healthier and digests your food better if it isn't!

Eat 20% fewer carbs. Carbs are an important part of a healthy balanced diet even for someone trying to lose weight, but you do need to eat them in moderation. Make sure then that your carb portion per meal is no bigger than the palm of your hand.

LOW–GI

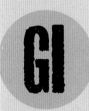

The Glycaemic Index (GI) is a measure of how quickly blood-sugar levels rise after eating a particular food. Foods with a high-GI, such as processed breads, grains and cereals and refined sugars, are broken down into glucose very quickly, which means they provide a fast energy fix and a rapid rise in blood-sugar levels. For anyone on a diet, this is not great news as it causes the release of insulin, which encourages the body to lay down fat. Foods with a low GI (less than 55) are absorbed more slowly and steadily into the bloodstream, helping you feel full for longer and making you less likely to want to snack. The recipes in *Skinny Weeks* all feature foods such as wholegrain carbs, green vegetables, fruits and lean protein that have a naturally low GI. These are all foods that I believe boost your metabolism, and encourage weight loss while also being kind to your heart and blood-sugar levels.

And remember, whether you're cooking from *Skinny Weeks* or not, make sure you're doing the following:

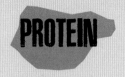

GET YOUR FILL OF PROTEIN

Protein helps you feel fuller for longer, making it an excellent choice for a dieter. As a result, the recipes within *Skinny Weeks* feature lots of lean proteins like low-fat dairy, lean red meat, chicken and fish. Other protein-rich food like nuts and seeds come combined with a hefty dose of fat. This doesn't make them a bad food or mean that you can't eat them on a diet – it simply means you need to keep an eye on portion sizes and keep them modest.

WATCH THE CARBS

We overeat our carbohydrate portions massively in this country, but really we should be eating between 50–80g of carbohydrates with each meal – this amounts to the equivalent of a slice of bread, 3–4 new potatoes or a handful of rice. This may sound mean, but it's all our bodies need. Eating protein with carbohydrates (adding tuna mayonnaise to a jacket potato, for example) helps lower the GI levels of the carbohydrates, making them less likely to be turned into sugar and then into fat.

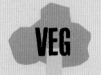

VEG OUT

Vegetables are fat-free, high in fibre and low in calories, which makes them a dieter's best friend. If you like to see a lot of food on your plate – go large on vegetables. It's very easy to get stuck in a rut buying same old veggies week in week out. Be adventurous. Each time you go to the supermarket or market pick up something new!

SUGAR

The most complex of foods; I believe that many of our health problems arise as a result of our consumption of refined sugars. In its natural forms, sugar contains a certain amount of fibre; however, when it is processed, this fibre is whipped away, leaving nothing to stop it being absorbed immediately into our blood stream. As a result, our blood sugar levels go wild, which puts demands on our livers and other organs, but also affects our glucose and insulin levels. I am not saying give up all the good sweet stuff, but merely consider the types of sugar you are eating. White refined sugars are the worst, but there are some sugars that are really mild and sit very low on the GI chart.

Here are some of my favourites:

Muscovado sugar: unrefined brown sugar with a wonderful flavour.

Rapadura sugar: a raw, unrefined toffee-ish cane sugar. The best everyday alternative to regular sugar.

Fructose: sweeter than regular sugar which means you need add less and it's relatively low-GI. Good for baking.

Agave nectar: produced from a cactus grown in South America. Agave syrup is about 30% sweeter than sugar or honey and has a GI between 11 and 19, depending on the brand. It tastes like a real sugar syrup, which is joy when most of the sugar-alternative syrups taste synthetic or ghastly.

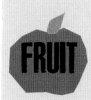

BE CLEVER WITH THE FRUIT

Fruits contain quite a bit of sugar but – because they also contain fibre, vitamins minerals and a whole host of phytochemicals – are great for you and should be eaten daily. Stick to 1 or 2 portions of fruit a day and try and eat your fruit whole and fresh, rather than in juice or smoothie form. Dried fruit does make a good snack but be careful about portion sizes (no more than 25g per snack). Eating a handful of nuts and seeds with fresh fruit helps lower its GI level and makes the body work harder to digest it.

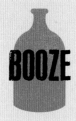

LOSE THE BOOZE

Alcohol is discouraged when dieting because it's full of calories and sugar. It's worth noting a bottle of wine has as many calories as a cheeseburger! If not drinking is not an option, then try to stick to white spirits like gin or vodka with a calorie-free mixer during the week and save that glass of wine for weekends.

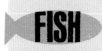

OPT FOR OILY FISH

Oily fish such as salmon, mackerel and sardines are rich in omega-3 fatty acids which can help reduce cholesterol and are fantastic for your heart, skin and joints. Nutritionists recommend that we should eat at least 2 portions of fish a week, 1 of which should be an oil-rich variety. Aim for a serving size of 100–125g per portion.

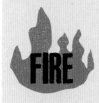

PICK FOODS THAT FIRE YOUR FURNACE

Okay, there are no quick fixes for dieting but it is true that some foods speed up your metabolism. Green tea, chillies, bio-yoghurt, cider vinegar and organic beef and dairy are all ingredients that can help give your metabolism a swift kick in the right direction, and all of them feature at some point or another during my *Skinny Weeks*.

GET MOVING

There's no escaping the fact that exercise and weight loss go hand in hand, so try and find some form of exercise that works for you and stick to it. Personally I run between 5–10k 3 times a week or do kettle bell or circuit training 2 or 3 times. Is it a bore? Well, yes it is sometimes, but I am so much better off for it. My brain works better, in that I can think clearer, I have less anxiety, and yes, it keeps me trim. What's not to like?

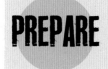

BE PREPARED

I hate to break it to you, but weight loss can be a bit like a job and it takes a little bit of elbow grease. The best advice I can give you when trying to slim down is to be prepared. This means everything from having your shopping done all the way through to making time to prepare your lunch and breakfast, not just your supper. Every Sunday night I do an online supermarket order for most of my bits. I use a butcher or fishmonger for my proteins. I then cook up in batches, making a vat of soup which will sort a few lunches during the week and mixing up my cereal by making either the Sunshine Bircher Muesli base (p22) or the Apple and Pecan Granola (p19). This leaves me only having to focus on cooking dinner from scratch and takes the pain out of the working week.

SKINNY WEEKS SURVIVAL TIPS...

1 Put all of the bad foods that you tend to snack on away. Out of sight, out of mind... If you see them, you are far more likely to want to eat them!

2 When you go out or your friends invite you round for dinner, scoff down the veggies, eat a normal portion of protein and leave half the carbohydrate they put on your plate. It's a good trick and how I manage.

3 Don't be afraid to use big flavours and high-fat ingredients like chorizo and Parmesan cheese in your cooking – just use them in small quantities. Team them up with low-calorie ingredients like white fish, fruit and veg, and chicken to give your food a big old flavour boost.

4 A well-stocked store cupboard is worth its weight in gold. For me, there are almost always aromatics like garlic, chilli, and ginger in the fridge, a spice cupboard filled to the rafters and tons of fresh herbs on the side. This means that even at a moment's notice I can rustle up a quick marinade, rub or herb sauce to put on a simple piece of meat or fish.

5 One of my favourite things to eat in a hurry is Chinese fried eggs with broccoli. Simply fry two eggs in a little oil, steam some tenderstem broccoli and top with the eggs. Douse with a tablespoon of oyster sauce and then top with a little chopped red chilli and spring onion. And there you have it. It takes 5 minutes, fills you up and tastes better than anything from the Chinese takeaway.

"SKINNY" WEEK

BREAKFASTS ON THE GO! * WORKING LUNCHES * SKINNY
DIPPING * SIMPLE SUPPERS * PUDS (IF YOU MUST...)

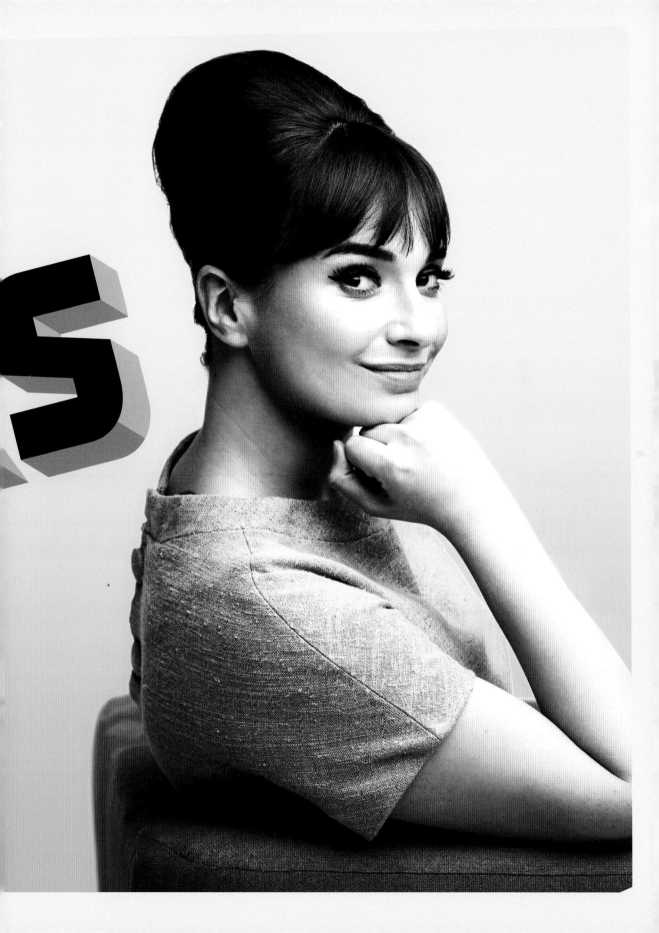

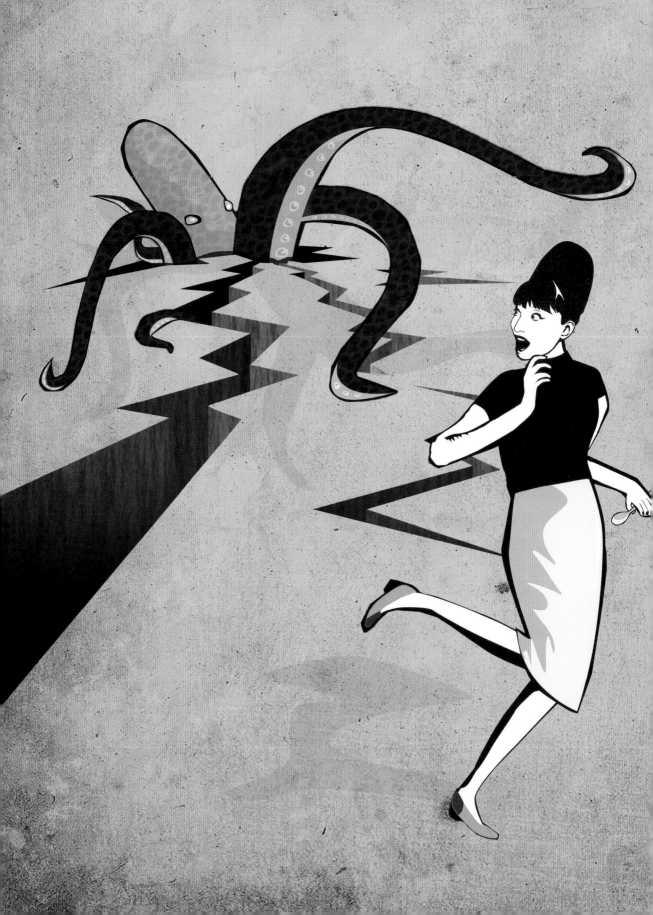

BREAKFASTS
on the go!

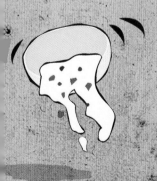

BANANA AND PEANUT BUTTER POWERSHAKE

Protein shakes are generally regarded as a bit of a culinary no-no, as on the whole, protein powders are pretty scary things. Nowadays, however, it is possible to get hold of really good-quality organic whey powder, which is packed full of the protein that will keep you feeling full. Mixed into smoothies or shakes, it makes a great quick breakfast.

1 small, very ripe banana,
   peeled and chopped
1 tbsp smooth peanut butter
1 tbsp flavourless organic whey
   protein powder (from good
   health food shops)
¼ tsp vanilla extract
250ml semi-skimmed milk
a glassful of ice

Put all of the ingredients into a blender and blitz for about 1 minute, or until everything is smooth.

 300 CALORIES

SERVES 1

PREPARATION TIME 5 MINUTES

MOCHA POWER SHAKE

My morning coffee is an integral part of my day, I'm ashamed to say that without it I am pretty much useless. All too often I find myself needing to leg it out of the door with only 5 minutes to drink coffee and eat breakfast. At such times this shake has become a lifesaver – giving me a bit of a chocolate fix and a big kick up the bum for the hectic day ahead.

1–2 shots of freshly
   brewed espresso
1 tsp good-quality cocoa powder
1 tsp agave nectar
1 tbsp flavourless organic whey
   protein powder (from good
   health food shops)
¼ tsp vanilla extract
200ml semi-skimmed milk
a glassful of ice

Put all of the ingredients into a blender and blitz for about 1 minute, or until everything is smooth.

 135 CALORIES

SERVES 1

PREPARATION TIME 5 MINUTES

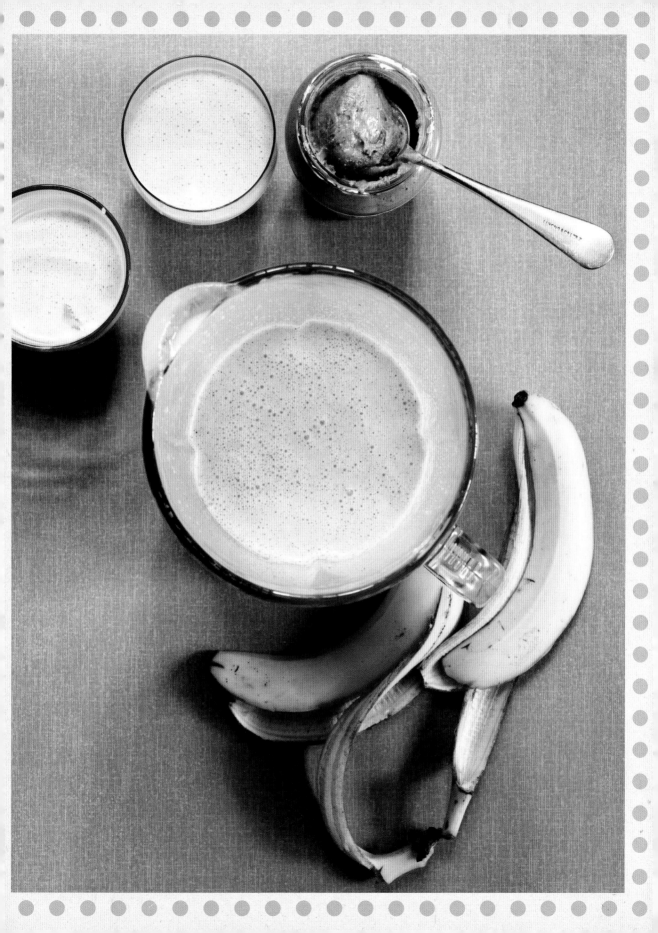

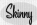
A BERRY GOOD START

This is my take on the 'magical breakfast cream' from the book *French Women Don't Get Fat*. A delicious way to start the day, it gives you a high-protein breakfast that is speedy to make and can be eaten on the go.

150g 0% fat Greek yoghurt
1 tsp flaxseed oil
50g old-fashioned oats
the juice and pulp of 2 clementines
a handful of mixed berries, mashed
    with **1 tsp agave nectar**
1 tbsp milled flaxseed, sunflower
    and pumpkin seeds

Mix the yoghurt and flaxseed oil together in a bowl. Pour over the oats, citrus juice and pulp and leave for a minute for the oats to soften. Stir in the berries and milled seeds and transfer to two serving bowls.

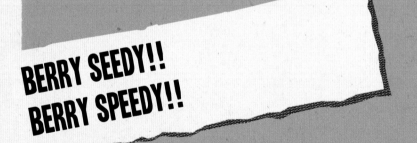

BERRY SEEDY!!
BERRY SPEEDY!!

216 CALORIES

PREPARATION TIME **5 MINUTES**

MAKES 2
PORTIONS

GIZZI TIP

If you've made up a batch of the rhubarb compote (p20) try substituting 3 tablespoons of it for the mixed berries.

★ ★ ★ ★ ★ ★ ★ ★ ★ ★ ★ ★ ★ ★ ★ ★ ★ ★ ★

APPLE, PECAN AND CINNAMON GRANOLA

Making your own granola may seem like a pointless faff, but you'd be shocked to see how much sugar and fat goes into the shop-bought ones. Besides, it's a rather nice way to spend a Sunday afternoon and it lasts for ages. This one's extra-special, inspired by apple crumble and made with dried apples, pecans and cinnamon. It's tremendous with milk or yoghurt and berries as a quick breakfast, or made into a posh – but equally as quick – rhubarb parfait (p20).

---

2 tbsp golden rapeseed oil
100ml agave nectar
1 tbsp honey
1 tsp cinnamon
1 tsp vanilla extract
300g muesli mix, with oats, spelt,
    rye (from health food stores)
25g sunflower seeds
25g pumpkin seeds
2 tbsp sesame seeds
75g pecans, roughly chopped
100g dried apple rings,
    roughly chopped

Preheat the oven to 150°C/Gas 2. Mix the oil, agave nectar, honey, cinnamon and vanilla in a large bowl. Tip in all the remaining ingredients except the apples and mix well. Pop the mix onto two baking sheets and spread evenly.

Bake for 20 minutes, then mix in the apples and bake for a further 10 minutes. Remove and scrape onto a flat tray to cool. Once cool, transfer to an airtight container until needed (the granola can be stored for up to a month).

To serve, put 75g of the granola in a bowl and cover with 3 tablespoons of cold semi-skimmed milk or fat-free yoghurt.

GRANOLA!

307 CALORIES

MAKES 10 PORTIONS

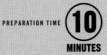

PREPARATION TIME 10 MINUTES

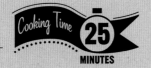

Cooking Time 25 MINUTES

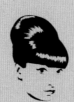

GIZZI TIP

I am using agave nectar, rapeseed oil and a multi-grain muesli mix here. Agave is one of the lowest-GI sugars on the market, while rapeseed gives the granola a buttery taste and is super healthy. The muesli includes a mix of different grains, meaning not only is it varied in flavour and super-delicious, but your body has to really work to burn it off.

★ ★ ★ ★ ★ ★ ★ ★ ★ ★ ★ ★ ★ ★ ★ ★ ★

RHUBARB COMPOTE AND GRANOLA PARFAIT

Rhubarb compote topped with low-fat yoghurt and homemade granola makes for quite the virtuous start to the day. I can't get enough of rhubarb, (I have a 'thing' for pink food) with its sweet/sour flavour. It makes the best compote around. Make a batch of this on the weekend and it'll last you the week. You'll then be able to have a breakfast that you would happily buy, in your own home, just by bunging a few things together every morning.

for the rhubarb compote
the juice of 2 oranges or apples
3 tbsp agave nectar
1 vanilla pod, split lengthways
1kg rhubarb, trimmed, washed and
    cut into 2cm chunks

for the parfait
2 tbsp 0% fat Greek yoghurt
2 tbsp Apple, Pecan and Cinnamon
    Granola (p19)

To make the compote, put the juice, agave nectar and vanilla pod in a pan over a low heat and stir until the agave nectar dissolves. Add the rhubarb and bring to a simmer, then remove from the heat. Cover and set aside for 10 minutes. The rhubarb pieces should break down into compote in that time. If not, cover for another 5 minutes, then remove the vanilla pod. Transfer to an airtight container and store in the fridge until needed (the compote will keep for up to 4 days).

To make the parfait, put 3 tablespoons of the compote into a dessert glass or jam jar. Top with the yoghurt and then the granola and serve.

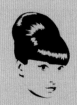 **GIZZI TIP**

This parfait also makes a great speedy pudding if you find yourself needing something sweet later in the day!

★ ★

173 CALORIES

PREPARATION TIME **5** MINUTES

MAKES 1
parfait/10
compote portions

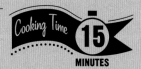 Cooking Time **15** MINUTES

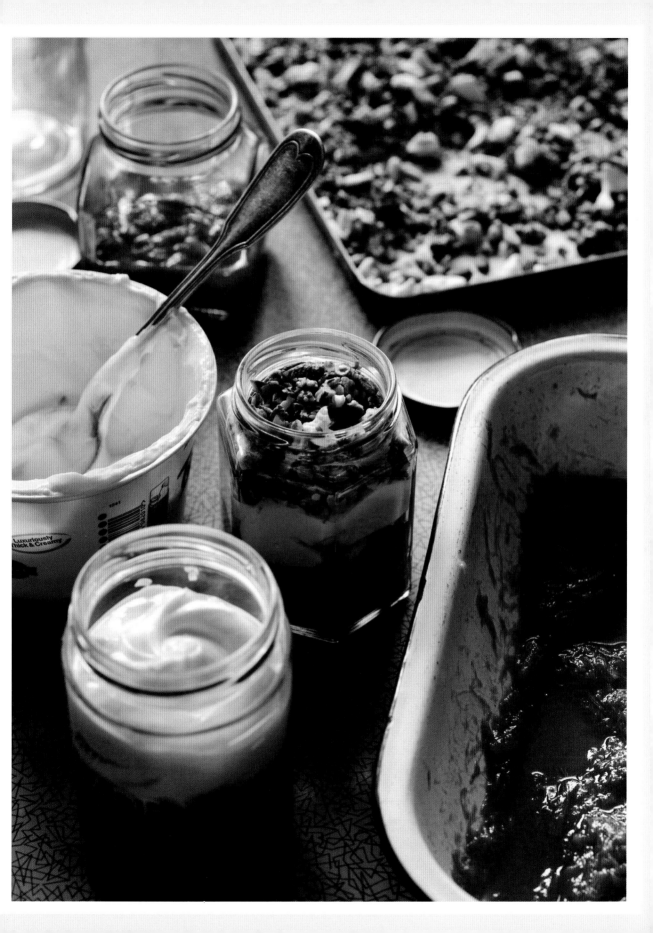

SUNNY BIRCHER MUESLI

Quick!

Bircher muesli combines dried fruits, nuts and oats that are soaked overnight with grated apple and milk. It was created by Dr Bircher-Benner in the 1890s for him to give to his patients in his Zurich clinic so they could face the day with optimum energy. He wasn't wrong – a bowl of this will have you cartwheeling down the halls. I've given this Bircher a tropical spin by using dried pineapple and mango, but noone is going to disapprove if you fancy staying traditional with raisins and sultanas instead.

for the main bulk
600g organic Scotch porridge oats
100g oat bran
100g dried pineapple, (the sugar-free stuff), chopped into raisin-sized pieces
100g dried mango, (the sugar-free stuff), chopped into raisin-sized pieces
50g unsweetened desiccated coconut
50g mixed nuts (e.g. Brazils, almonds, hazelnuts), toasted, then roughly chopped
50g milled flaxseed, sunflower and pumpkin seeds

for bringing to life
1 apple, grated
200ml semi-skimmed milk, plus extra for serving
a handful of raspberries and blueberries

Pop all the main bulk ingredients into one of those great sealable plastic cereal boxes and shake wildly until all the different ingredients have been blended together. The muesli can be stored for up to 2 months.

To make your bircher for the following day, put the grated apple, milk and 200g of the bulk mix in a bowl and stir immediately, so that the apple doesn't have a chance to go brown. Cover with clingfilm and pop in the fridge overnight.

The next morning, split the soaked muesli between two bowls and serve with the berries and 30ml milk per portion.

338 CALORIES

MAKES 2 bowls of Bircher muesli/20 main bulk portions

PREPARATION TIME **10 MINUTES** (plus overnight soaking)

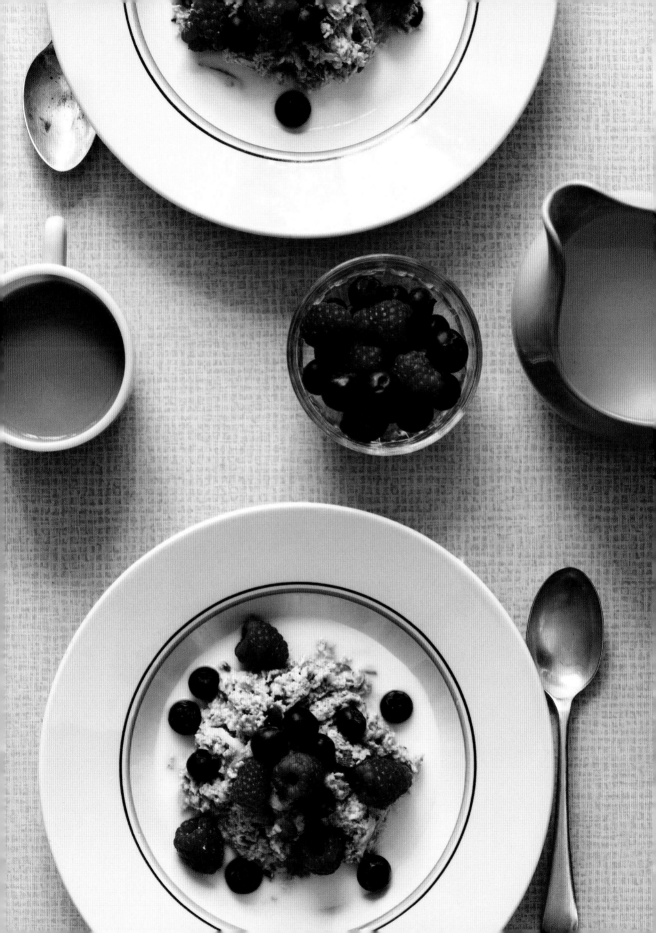

SEEDY DIPPY EGGS WITH MARMITE SOLDIERS

I've been scraping Marmite on my toast with eggs since I was a nipper. It adds seasoning and an umami roundness (the so called 'fifth taste', which makes certain savoury foods uniquely satisfying) to it. I now feel short-changed without it. If you have never done this before I insist you try it.

---

sea salt
1 large free-range egg
1 thin slice of sourdough bread
a knob of butter
a scraping of Marmite
1 tbsp mixed seeds

Bring a small pan of salted water to a simmer. Add the egg and simmer for 4 minutes and 20 seconds. (Yes, I know: this is very exact but it will guarantee a perfectly boiled egg!).

Meanwhile, toast the bread and spread thinly with the butter, then the Marmite. Cut the toast into soldiers. Dip each into the egg, scatter over a few mixed seeds and eat.

'Boiled Alive!!'

 300 CALORIES

PREPARATION TIME **1** MINUTE

SERVES 1

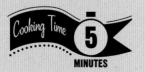 Cooking Time **5** MINUTES

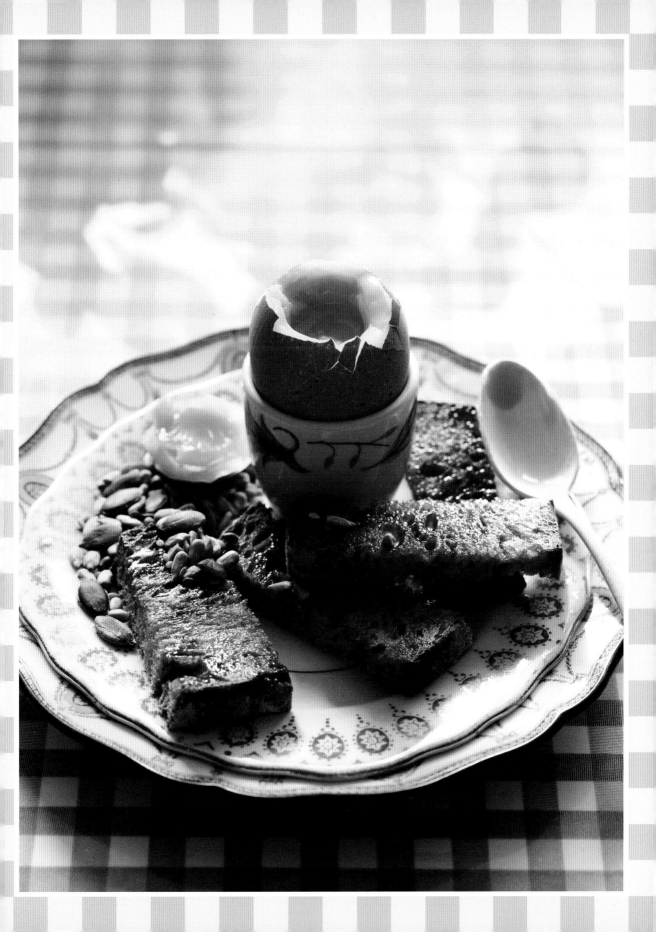

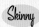

AVOCADO ON TOAST

The Breakfast of Kings... I need say no more.

---

1 small ripe avocado
juice of ½ a lemon
1 thin slice of sourdough
    bread, toasted
sea salt and freshly ground
    black pepper
½ **red chilli,** deseeded and finely
    chopped (if you're feeling like
    some spice)

Halve your avocado and remove the stone. Squeeze a little lemon juice on the cut surface of one half, wrap in clingfilm and pop in the fridge to be eaten as soon as possible.

Scoop the flesh out of the remaining half and pile it on top of your toast. Mash it down a little with a fork, squeeze over a little more lemon juice, season with salt and pepper and sprinkle over the chopped chilli, if using.

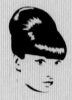

GIZZI TIP

If you have a little time on your hands, try griddling your bread on a dry, hot griddle pan for extra smoky flavour.

★ ★ ★ ★ ★ ★ ★ ★ ★ ★ ★ ★ ★ ★ ★ ★ ★

278 CALORIES

PREPARATION TIME
5 MINUTES

SERVES 1

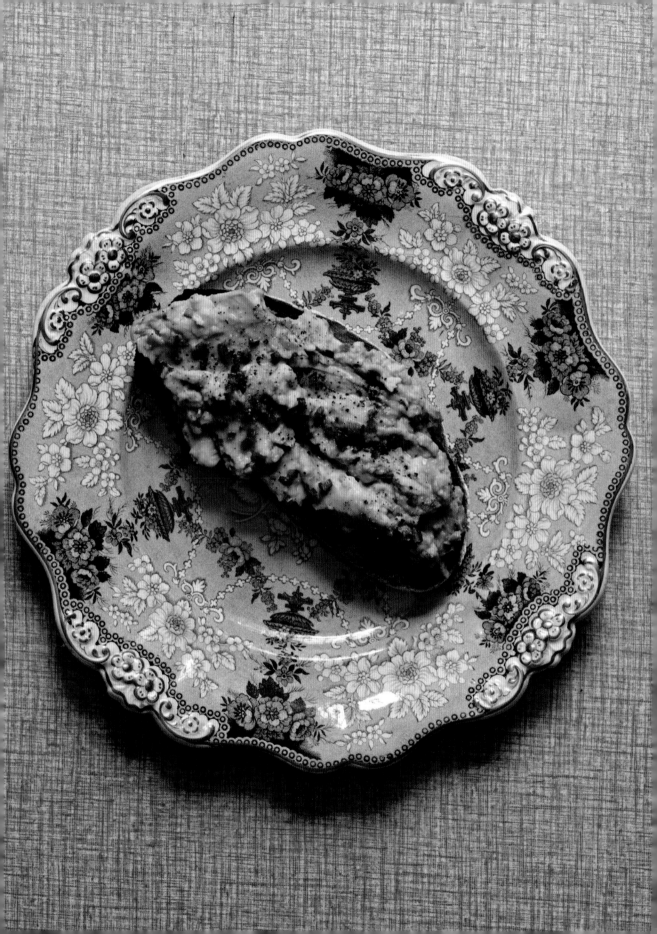

ELVIS TOASTS

Elvis loved his peanut butter and banana sandwiches and myth states that he actually died on the loo eating one. His were fried, though, making them a massive 2000 calories each. I'm doing them virtuously here on toasted sourdough, a spreading of chunky peanut butter and some sliced banana. Heaven, but also the ultimate power breakfast.

1 thin slice of sourdough rye bread
1 ½ tbsp crunchy peanut butter
½ banana, sliced
1 small cube of good-quality dark chocolate (70% cocoa solids)

Lightly toast the bread. While it's still hot, spread it with the peanut butter. Lay on the slices of banana, grate over the chocolate and munch.

 284 CALORIES   SERVES 1   PREPARATION TIME **5** MINUTES

BACON, AVOCADO AND TOMATO ON RYE

There are some days when you just **need** a bacon sandwich. I know, I have many of them. What you might not realise, though, is that bacon can be less fattening than eating cereal, so don't feel like you can't eat it. It's how you do so that matters. Trimming the bacon means you wave goodbye to two-thirds of the calories, helping move this open sarnie into skinny territory.

2 rashers of smoked bacon, trimmed of fat
15g low-fat cream cheese
1 thin slice of seeded rye sourdough, toasted
½ small ripe avocado, sliced
a squeeze of lemon juice
sea salt and freshly ground black pepper
1 tomato, sliced

Heat the griddle pan to smoking, add the bacon and cook for 1–2 minutes on each side until cooked through and slightly charred. Spread the cream cheese over the bread.

Mash the avocado in a bowl, add the lemon juice and season with salt and pepper. Arrange over the bread and top with the bacon and sliced tomato. Serve hot.

310 CALORIES   SERVES 1   PREPARATION TIME **10** MINUTES   Cooking Time **5** MINUTES

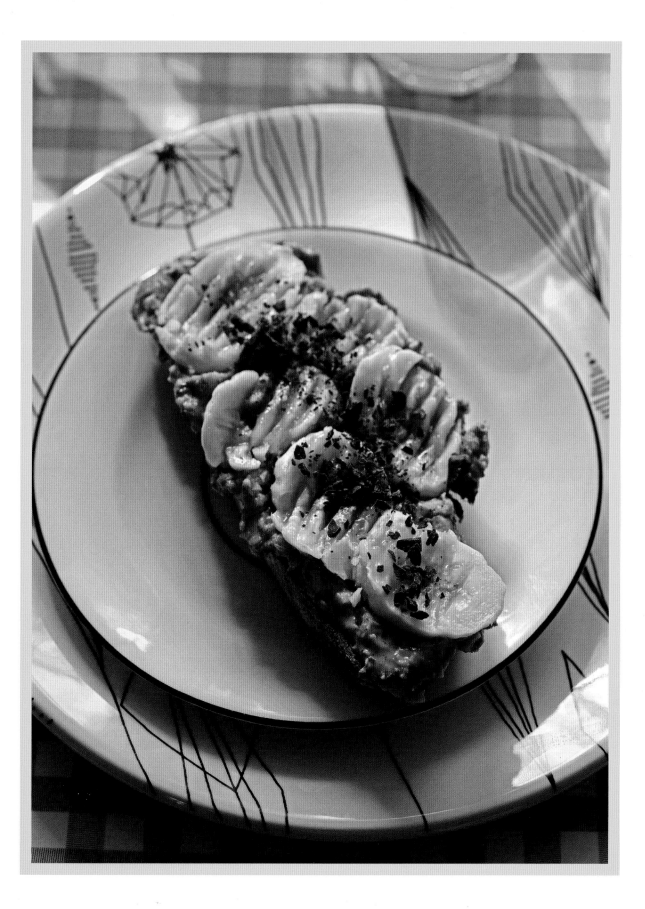

GRILLED TOMATOES ON TOAST WITH CREME FRAICHE AND FLOWERING MARJORAM

Fat grilled tomatoes turned through crème fraîche are one of life's little pleasures. They remind me of my father, though his preference would have been for plum tomatoes in juice over fresh grilled ones. A generational thing, I think...

2 medium vine-ripened tomatoes, halved
1 tsp good extra-virgin olive oil
sea salt and freshly ground black pepper
½ tsp fresh marjoram flowers or dried marjoram leaves
1 thin slice of sourdough bread
1 tbsp half-fat crème fraîche

Preheat the grill to high. Rub the tomato halves with half the oil, season with salt and pepper and scatter over the marjoram. Cook under the hot grill for 5–7 minutes, until softened.

Meanwhile, toast or griddle the bread and drizzle with the rest of the oil.

Stir the grilled tomatoes gently through the crème fraîche. Use to top the toast, squashing them slightly so the juices soak into the bread.

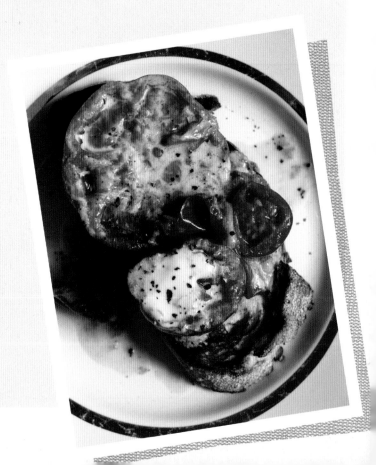

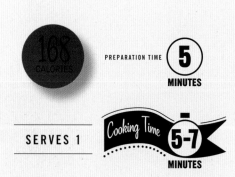

168 CALORIES

PREPARATION TIME **5** MINUTES

SERVES 1

Cooking Time **5-7** MINUTES

MUSHROOMS ON TOAST

This is a right meaty plateful of food that will leave you full for ages. Some people may think I'm crazy eating garlic for breakfast – if you do, then leave it out. But if it's flavour you're after then leave it in – it's delicious! I also love this for supper when I really cannot be bothered to cook.

2 tsp olive oil
100g chestnut mushrooms, sliced
100g field or portobello
    mushrooms, sliced
1–2 garlic cloves, finely chopped
1 tbsp half-fat crème fraîche
½ tsp chopped parsley
zest of ½ a lemon
sea salt and freshly ground
    black pepper
2 thin slices of sourdough
    bread, toasted

Heat a small frying pan until really hot, then add the oil and mushrooms and stir-fry on a high heat for 3–4 minutes, or until browned. (You're looking for nicely browned mushrooms that are frying dryly – if the mushrooms release water then the pan is not hot enough!) Add the garlic and continue to fry for another minute or two.

Stir through the crème fraîche, parsley and lemon zest and season with salt and pepper. Spoon the mushrooms over the toast and serve.

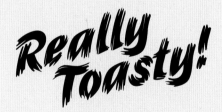

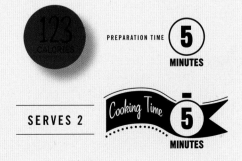

123 CALORIES

PREPARATION TIME **5** MINUTES

SERVES 2

Cooking Time **5** MINUTES

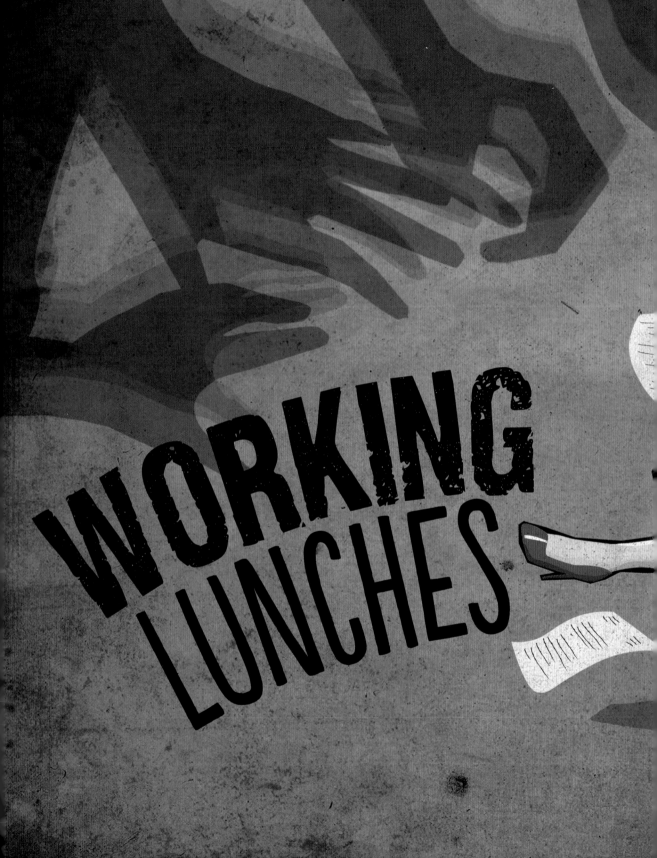

WORKING
LUNCHES

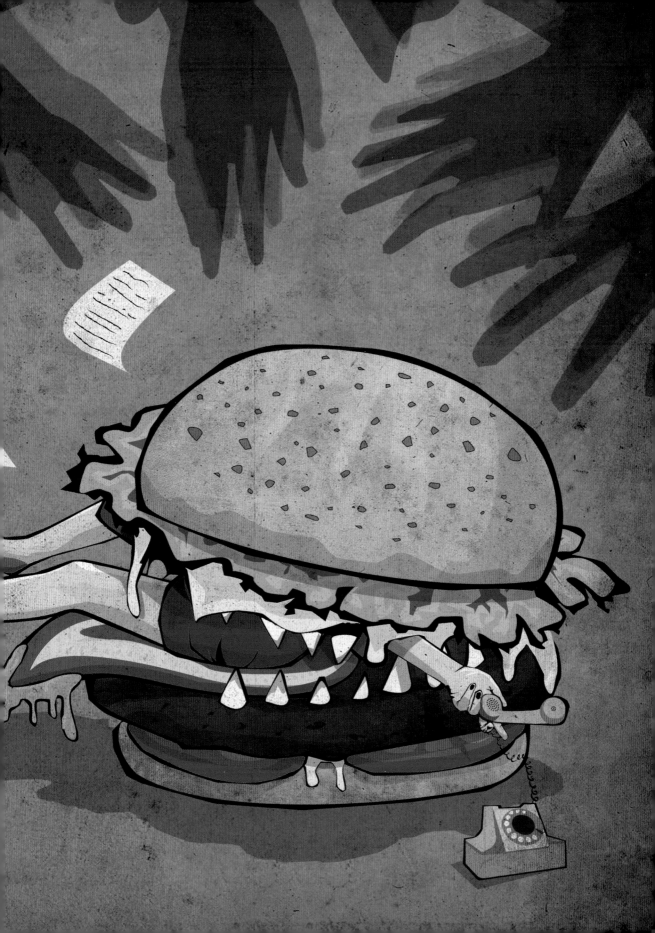

SALADE TROPICALE

This is about as retro as a salad can get. Classically the hearts of palm, papaya and avocado would be tossed with bib lettuce, but I've added my favourite beach food, sea bass ceviche, to the mix. Ceviche is a way of 'cooking' fish by marinating it in lime juice and salt, though it still retains its rawness in the centre. It is fresh, zingy and super-healthy.

200g super-fresh sea bass, filleted and skinned in one piece if possible

1 small red onion, finely chopped

1 small garlic clove, grated

1 red chilli, finely sliced

1 tsp sea salt

juice of 3 limes

a good handful of fresh coriander, finely chopped

1–2 tomatoes, deseeded and finely chopped

5 radishes, thinly sliced

1 x 400g can palm hearts, sliced into rounds, (optional)

1 medium ripe but firm avocado, peeled, stoned and chopped

1 papaya, peeled, deseeded and chopped

1 tbsp really good-quality extra-virgin olive oil

Lay the sea bass on a chopping board and slice it into pieces about 5mm thick. Pop the fish in a bowl with the onion, garlic, chilli, salt, lime juice and coriander and mix well. Cover with clingfilm and put in the fridge for 20 minutes, giving it a stir halfway through.

Add the tomatoes, radishes, palm hearts, avocado, papaya and oil to the marinated fish and mix with your hands until combined. Divide between bowls to serve.

377 CALORIES

PREPARATION TIME **15 MINUTES**

SERVES 2

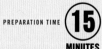 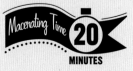

Macerating Time **20 MINUTES**

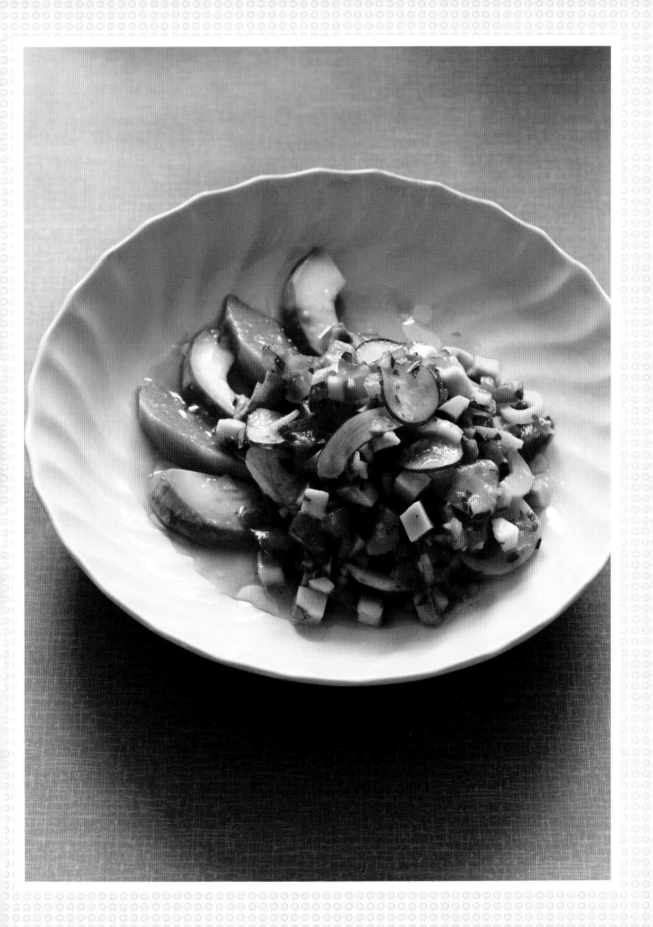

CHOPPED SALAD WITH BACON AND BLUE CHEESE

Salad culture in California is a big deal and those West-siders make some of the best salads around, as they aren't afraid to use bold flavours and interesting techniques. The most famous salad there has to be the simple chopped salad, which differs from place to place. So what's a chopped salad? It's a salad that's been chopped so all the ingredients are around the same size, making it easy to get a bit of everything into each mouthful. With ingredients such as blue cheese, bacon and eggs, this salad is an orgasmic mix of colours, textures and flavours.

2 free-range eggs
4 rashers of smoked back bacon, fat trimmed
1 head of romaine lettuce
2 vine-ripened tomatoes
1 small ripe avocado
1 cooked beetroot
40g blue cheese, crumbled (Stilton or Gorgonzola are great)
30ml base dressing (see below)

Hard-boil the eggs for 7 minutes, before peeling them under running cold water. Gently heat a non-stick frying pan, add the bacon and cook over a low heat for about 5 minutes, or until the bottom has turned crisp and golden. Using a fish slice, flip it over carefully and cook the other side for 5 minutes, or until the fat has rendered (you should be left with a good couple of teaspoons in the pan) and the bacon is nicely crisp. Drain the bacon on kitchen paper, then chop or crumble into bite-sized pieces.

On a large wooden board, separately chop the lettuce, tomatoes, avocado, beetroot and eggs into bite-sized pieces, then combine the ingredients and continue chopping and mixing together. Add the cheese and bacon, pour over the dressing and give everything a final mix. Divide between plates to serve.

BASE DRESSING

Pop 100ml really good-quality extra-virgin olive oil, 3 tbsp red-wine vinegar, 1 tbsp lemon juice, 1 tsp Dijon mustard and a little salt and pepper in a small bowl and whisk until combined. Alternatively, throw all the ingredients into a clean jam jar, place the lid on tightly and shake like a mad thing. Store either in or out of the fridge and use within a week (1 tablespoon = 61 calories).

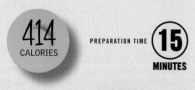

414 CALORIES

PREPARATION TIME **15** MINUTES

SERVES 2

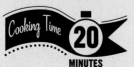
Cooking Time **20** MINUTES

CRUNCHY TUNA SALAD WITH EGG

This salad is staple Erskine fodder – really easy and filling, with tons of texture, colour and simple flavours. It has hints of salad niçoise to it but is just a whole lot more energetic. I would always make sure the eggs are a bit gooey in the middle, so if you're planning to take this one to work, leave your eggs whole, then cut them in half when you're ready to eat it.

sea salt and freshly ground
  black pepper
2 free-range eggs
4 spring onions, finely chopped
1 celery stalk, chopped
8 radishes, quartered
1 red pepper, chopped
1 yellow or orange pepper, chopped
1 Lebanese cucumber or ½ regular
  cucumber, deseeded and chopped
1 little gem lettuce, washed, dried
  and finely chopped
1 x 170g can skipjack tuna
  in spring water, drained
40ml Base Dressing (see opposite)
juice of ½ a lemon

Bring a pan of salted water to the boil, add the eggs and cook for exactly 6 minutes (this will give you the perfect gooey-middled eggs). Remove from the water, drain and peel under cold, running water.

Put the chopped veg in a big mixing bowl, add the tuna, salad dressing and lemon juice and season with salt and pepper. Give everything a really good mix together and then split between 2 plates.

Halve the eggs lengthways through the yolks. Place 2 egg halves on top of each portion and serve.

340 CALORIES

PREPARATION TIME (15) MINUTES

SERVES 2

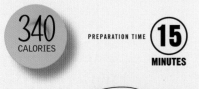 Cooking Time (6) MINUTES

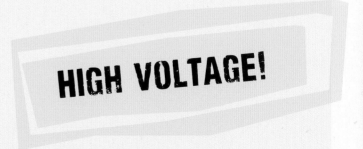 HIGH VOLTAGE!

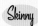

A NICE LITTLE SMOKED SALMON PLATE

This is the only way to describe this great little lunch. A plate of smoked salmon with all the trimmings, it's packed full of protein and simply leaves you with the biggest spring in your step. If you don't want to use any of the 'other bits' then leave them out, but frankly, I love them all.

---

2 quail's eggs
1 thin slice of sourdough bread
125g really good-quality cold-smoked salmon, cut into thin slices
1 small cooked beetroot, cut into small cubes
5 caper berries (in vinegar)
1 tbsp half-fat sour cream
1 tbsp salmon roe
a few sprigs of dill
a squeeze of lemon juice, plus a few wedges to serve
a good grinding of black pepper

Soft-boil the quail's eggs in boiling water for 2 ½ minutes. Peel and halve. Toast or griddle the bread.

Lay the smoked salmon in the centre of a plate. Arrange the beetroot, berries, sour cream, salmon roe, and quail's eggs over the salmon (you don't need to be too fussy about how you do this). Scatter over the dill, squeeze over the lemon juice and grind over a little black pepper to finish.

375 CALORIES

PREPARATION TIME 5

SERVES 1

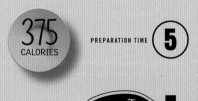 Cooking Time **5 MINUTES**

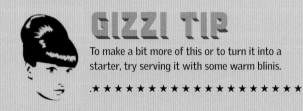 **GIZZI TIP**
To make a bit more of this or to turn it into a starter, try serving it with some warm blinis.

★ ★ ★ ★ ★ ★ ★ ★ ★ ★ ★ ★ ★ ★ ★ ★ ★ ★ ★

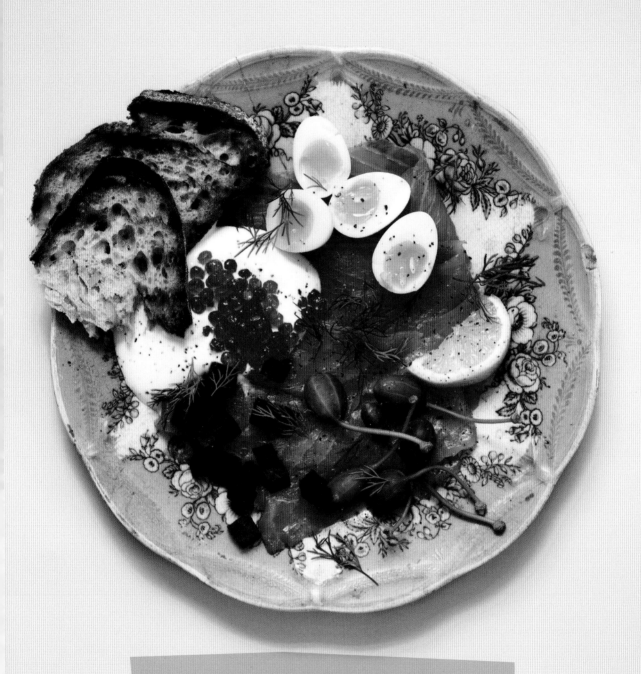

SMOKING!!!

RARE BEEF, POTATO, RADISH AND TOMATO SALAD

This salad screams summer to me. It's full of flavours that fit so perfectly with beef – horseradish, radishes, watercress, tomatoes – all thrown together to make a stylish little lunch.

1 tbsp olive oil

2 x 200g fillet steaks, each 5cm thick (or you could use leftover rare roast beef)

sea salt and freshly ground black pepper

100g half-fat crème fraîche

2 tbsp good-quality horseradish sauce

1 tbsp mayonnaise

300g Charlotte or other small waxy potatoes, cooked whole then cut in half lengthways

4 spring onions, thinly sliced

10 radishes, quartered

4 chives, snipped

200g mixed coloured heirloom tomatoes, sliced

1 bunch of watercress, trimmed

Heat the oil in a frying pan until really hot. Season the steaks with salt and pepper, then add to the pan and fry for 1 minute on each side, until the meat is brown on the outside but still rare in the middle. Remove from the pan and leave to cool, then wrap in clingfilm, transfer to the freezer and leave to rest for 1 hour, until the meat firms up and is almost frozen (a restaurant trick that will make it easier to slice).

Using a very sharp knife, thinly slice each steak into 12 slices. Mix the crème fraîche, horseradish and mayonnaise together in a bowl and season with salt and pepper. Add the potatoes, spring onions, radishes and chives and mix thoroughly. Divide the beef slices among 4 plates. Scatter over the tomatoes, then top with the potato mixture and watercress. Serve.

PREPARATION TIME **10** MINUTES

COOLING TIME **1** HOUR

SERVES 4

Cooking Time **2** MINUTES

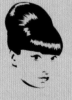

GIZZI TIP

This salad is just as good made with beef left over from the Sunday roast.

★ ★ ★ ★ ★ ★ ★ ★ ★ ★ ★ ★ ★ ★ ★ ★ ★

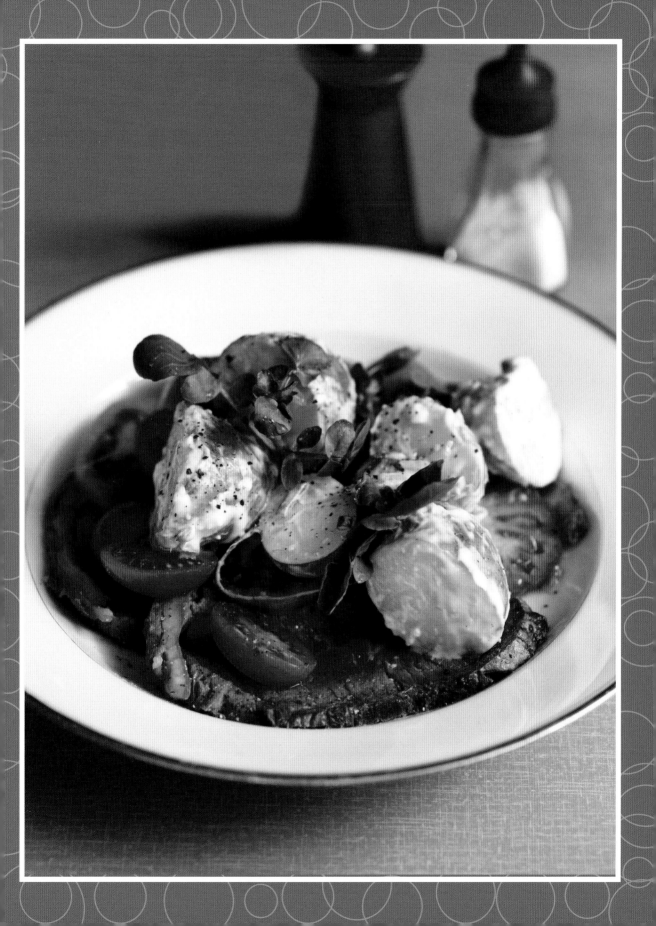

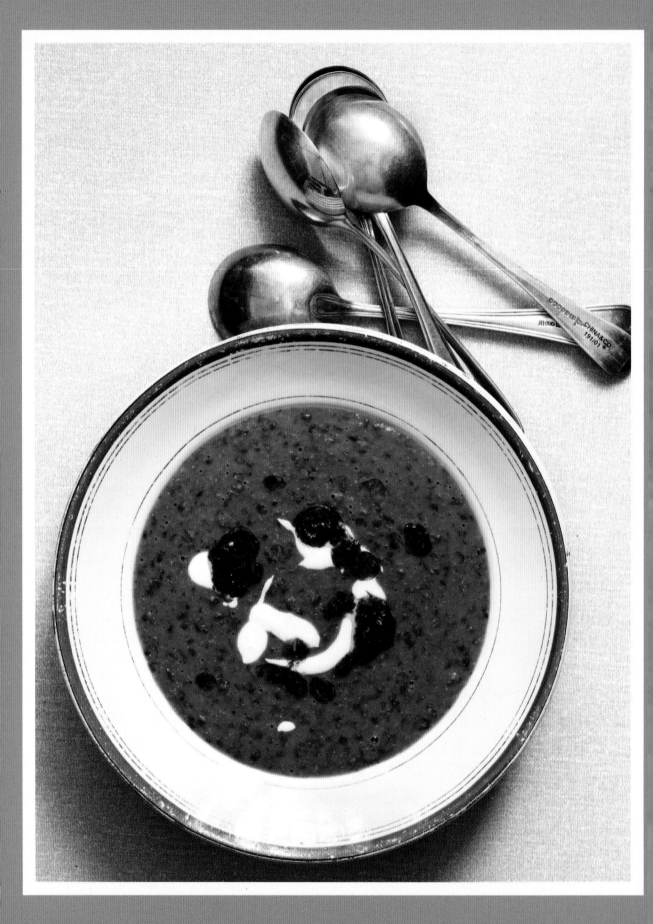

EGYPTIAN BLACK LENTIL SOUP WITH GREEN SAUCE

Black lentils are a beautiful ingredient full of energy-giving properties, which give body to soups and stews. This is not the classic Middle Eastern/Indian soup in that it's only mildly spiced, but the fragrant green sauce it's served with adds a mighty whack of POW to the proceedings. A splendid little lunch that will have you running rings round all your friends.

500g black (urad) lentils, washed
  and well drained
1 vine-ripened tomato, quartered
1 carrot, quartered
1 leek, quartered
2 large onions, 1 quartered and
  1 chopped
1.5 litres water
1 tbsp olive oil
2 garlic cloves, chopped
1 tbsp ground cumin
1 tsp sea salt
2 tbsp lime juice
0% fat Greek yoghurt, to serve

for the green sauce
1 small garlic clove
a small handful of parsley,
  roughly chopped
a small handful of mint,
  roughly chopped
3 tbsp olive oil
juice of ½ a lemon
**sea salt and freshly ground
  black pepper**

Put the lentils in a large pot, add the tomato, carrot, leek, quartered onion and water. Bring to the boil and then reduce to a simmer for 30 minutes.

Meanwhile, heat the oil in a large pot and fry the chopped onion for 7–8 minutes until softened and golden brown. Add the garlic and cumin and cook for a further 1–2 minutes, then add the sea salt and lime juice and simmer for a further 20 minutes, or until the lentils are soft (you may also need to add a little more water at this point if the lentils look like they are drying out). Pop the lentil and vegetable mix into a food processor and blitz until you have a fairly smooth soup, adding more water if necessary.

To make the green sauce, put all the ingredients into a pestle and mortar and pound together to form a coarse, chunky paste.

Put the soup back in the pan and reheat until piping hot, then pour into bowls. Top each bowl with a tablespoon each of the green sauce and yoghurt.

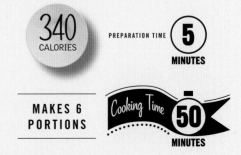

340 CALORIES

PREPARATION TIME (5) MINUTES

MAKES 6 PORTIONS

Cooking Time 50 MINUTES

CARROT AND LENTIL SOUP

This was one of the first soups I ever made when I got my fresh-out-of-catering-school arse onto BBC Good Food magazine. It's got everything you could ask for: delicious sweetness from the carrots, body from the lentils and tons of flavour from the spices, plus it's the easiest soup to make in history. I've been making it ever since.

---

1 tbsp cumin seeds
a large pinch of chilli flakes
1 tbsp olive oil
1kg carrots, washed and
    coarsely grated
200g split red lentils
1.5 litres chicken or vegetable stock
150ml semi-skimmed milk
0% fat Greek yoghurt, to serve
sea salt and freshly ground
    black pepper

for the coriander oil
a small bunch of coriander,
    roughly chopped
2 tbsp olive oil
zest and juice of 1 lime

Heat a large saucepan, add the cumin seeds and chilli flakes and dry-fry for 1 minute, or until they start to jump around the pan and release their aromas. Scoop out about half of the seeds with a spoon and set aside. Add the oil, carrot and lentils to the pan and sauté for 5 minutes, until the carrot has started to soften. Add the stock and bring to the boil. Reduce the heat and simmer for 15 minutes, until the lentils have swollen and softened, then add the milk. Cook for another 5 minutes before whizzing with a stick blender or in a food processor until smooth (or leave it chunky if you prefer). Season with salt and pepper.

To make the oil, put the chopped coriander in a pestle. Bash with the mortar to form a coarse paste, then add the oil, lime zest and juice and season to taste.

Portion the soup and serve with a tablespoon of yoghurt, a drizzle of the coriander oil and a sprinkling of the reserved toasted spices.

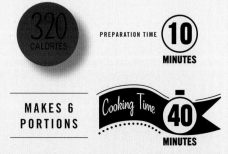

320 CALORIES

PREPARATION TIME **10** MINUTES

MAKES 6 PORTIONS

Cooking Time **40** MINUTES

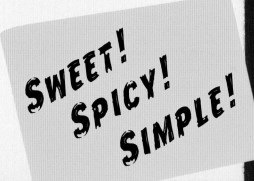

SWEET! SPICY! SIMPLE!

CHORIZO AND CHICKPEA SOUP WITH ROSE PETAL HARISSA

Chorizo makes everything taste amazing: it's a culinary fact. And it doesn't just work with Spanish flavours – it's great teamed with Northern African ones, too. The saffron, cumin, chilli and harissa make this wonderfully comforting soup a melting pot of massive flavours.

2 x 80g semi-cured chorizo sausages, chopped
1 onion, finely chopped
2 celery stalks, finely chopped
1 leek, finely chopped
1 carrot, peeled and finely chopped
3 garlic cloves, grated
1 bay leaf
a pinch of red chilli
½ tsp ground cumin
¼ tsp ground coriander
1 tbsp tomato purée
1 x 400g can of chopped tomatoes
1 litre chicken stock
1 x 400g can of chickpeas
a pinch of saffron (optional)
a small bunch of fresh coriander, chopped
a squeeze of lemon juice
sea salt and freshly ground black pepper
0% fat Greek yoghurt, to serve
rose petal harissa, to serve

Gently heat the chorizo in a large pan until it has released all its oil and has coloured slightly. Turn up the heat to high and fry for a further 2 minutes, until golden. (Chorizo is really fatty and if you are clever you can get those two sausages to release about 4–5 tablespoons of fat.) Drain off and discard as much of the fat as you can, leaving about 1 teaspoon in the pan.

Add the onion, celery, leek and carrot to the pan, lower the heat and gently fry for about 7 minutes, until the veg are slightly softened but not coloured. Add the garlic, bay leaf, chilli, cumin and coriander and cook for 1 minute, then add the tomato purée and cook, stirring to combine, for another minute. Add the tomatoes, stock, chickpeas, saffron (if using) and half the fresh coriander, bring to the boil, then leave to simmer gently for 20 minutes. Stir in the lemon juice and season to taste with salt and pepper. Serve the soup in bowls, topping each with a tablespoon of yoghurt, half a tablespoon of harissa and the remaining fresh coriander.

200 CALORIES

PREPARATION TIME (15) MINUTES

MAKES 6 PORTIONS

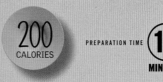

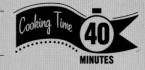

Cooking Time (40) MINUTES

PANCETTA, FARRO AND BEAN SOUP

A delish high-energy soup, which can be made in vats and bought to work to heat up, and will keep you fuller for longer. It's the sort of food I'd make for supper on a Sunday night, then portion the rest for work.

100g cubed pancetta
(or smoked bacon)
1 tbsp olive oil
1 bay leaf
1 onion, finely chopped
2 small carrots, peeled and
finely chopped
2 celery stalks, finely chopped
1 garlic clove, finely chopped
3 tomatoes, skinned, deseeded
and diced
1 tbsp tomato purée
1.5 litres chicken stock (fresh if you
can find it)
140g farro (pearled spelt) or pearl
barley, rinsed and drained
1 x 400g can of cannellini beans,
rinsed and drained
**sea salt and freshly ground
black pepper**
**a handful of chopped flat-leaf
parsley**, to serve
**10g freshly grated Parmesan
per person**, to serve

Fry the pancetta in the oil for 2–3 minutes in a large saucepan. Add the bay leaf, onion, carrot, and celery and cook over a gentle heat until the onion has softened and is starting to go golden, about 5 minutes. Add the garlic, fry for a minute more, then add the tomatoes and the tomato purée. Cook these down for 5 minutes, until the tomatoes start to thicken and soften.

Pour over the stock and bring to the boil. Add the drained farro to the stock, then simmer very gently for 25–30 minutes, until brothy and slightly reduced. Add the cannellini beans and simmer for a further 10 minutes, or until the grains are tender. Season with salt and freshly ground pepper. Ladle the soup into bowls, sprinkle over the parsley and Parmesan and serve.

ALWAYS ON A SUNDAY!

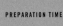
316 CALORIES

PREPARATION TIME **20** MINUTES

MAKES 6 PORTIONS

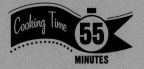
Cooking Time **55** MINUTES

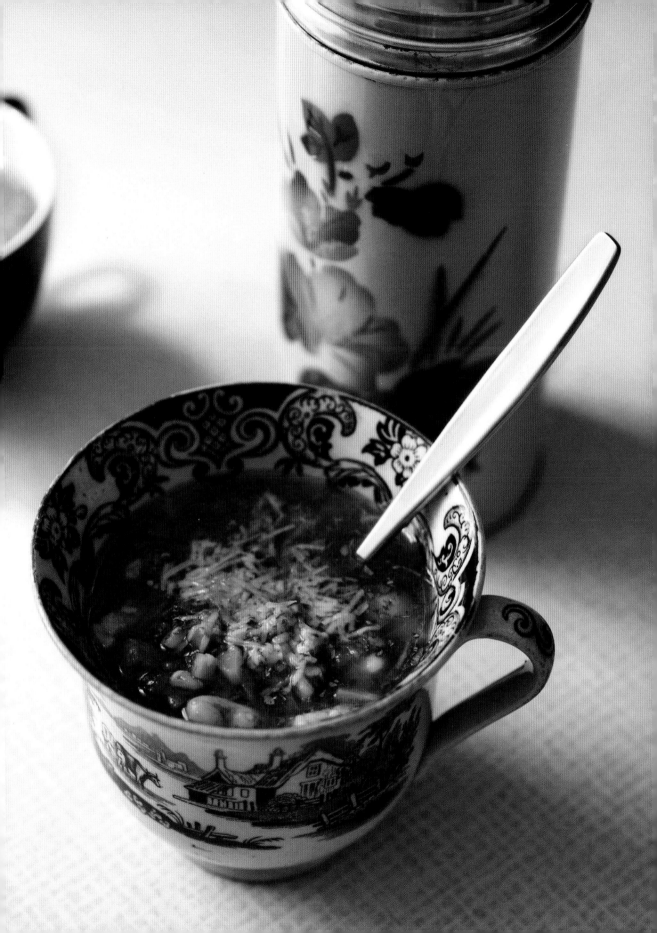

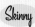
PERSIAN CHICKEN, BARLEY AND LEMON SOUP (ASH-E-JOW)

My friend Sabrina Ghayour is Persian and proud. She runs Persian and Middle Eastern supper clubs around London and is building up quite a reputation as one of the dons of Middle Eastern cooking. This soup of hers – the Persian answer to chicken noodle soup (aka Jewish penicillin) – has tons of flavour, is extremely satisfying and is really simple to make.

3 tbsp rapeseed or olive oil

4 free-range chicken thighs or legs
    on the bone

2 large onions, peeled and chopped

3 garlic cloves, finely chopped

1 tsp turmeric

175g barley

75g green lentils

sea salt and freshly ground
    black pepper

2 litres water

600ml chicken stock (fresh is best)

1 small bunch of fresh parsley

1 small bunch of fresh coriander

50g fresh spinach leaves

2 tbsp liquid whey (kashk)
    or 3 tbsp 0% fat Greek yoghurt

zest and juice of 1 small lemon

Heat half the oil in a large cooking pot over a medium to high heat. Add the chicken pieces and brown all over, then remove from the pan and set aside. Add the rest of the oil and the onions and sauté for 10 minutes, until the onions are softened and lightly brown. Add the garlic and turmeric and fry for a further minute, then add the chicken, barley and lentils to the pot and season well with salt and pepper. Cook for a few minutes, stirring, then add the water and stock and bring to the boil. Reduce the heat to low, cover and leave to simmer, stirring occasionally, for 45 minutes.

Remove the chicken from the pot and shred the meat from the bone. Return the shredded meat to the pot with the fresh herbs, spinach and the liquid whey or yoghurt and bring back to the boil. Stir in the lemon juice and zest, season with salt and pepper and ladle into bowls.

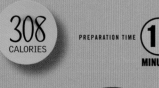

308 CALORIES

PREPARATION TIME (10) MINUTES

MAKES 6 PORTIONS

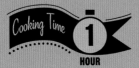

Cooking Time **(1)** HOUR

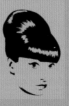

GIZZI TIP

Though this is delicious as it is for a simple, everyday lunch, to make it more special try topping it with its traditional garnish. Just add a few caramelised onions, a sprinkling of dried mint and a dash of turmeric powder along with a little extra liquid whey.

.★ ★ ★ ★ ★ ★ ★ ★ ★ ★ ★ ★ ★ ★ ★ ★ ★ ★ ★

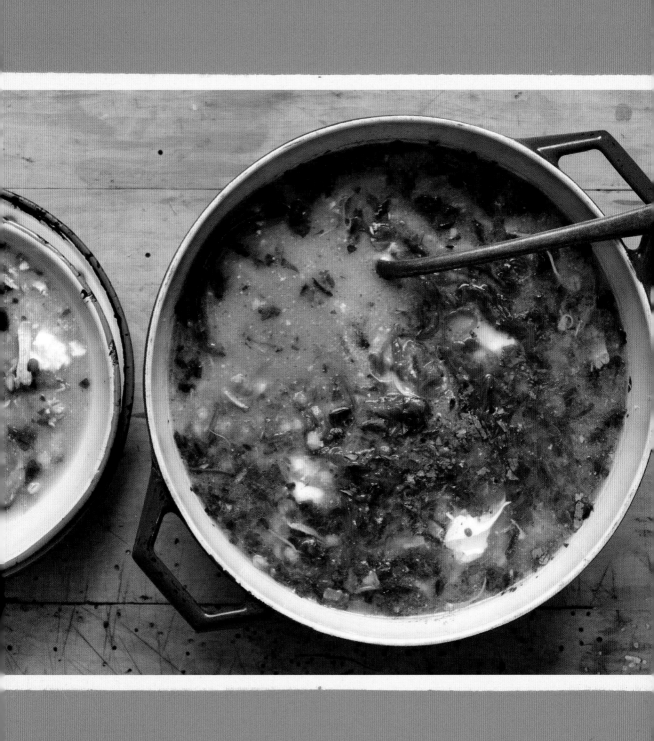

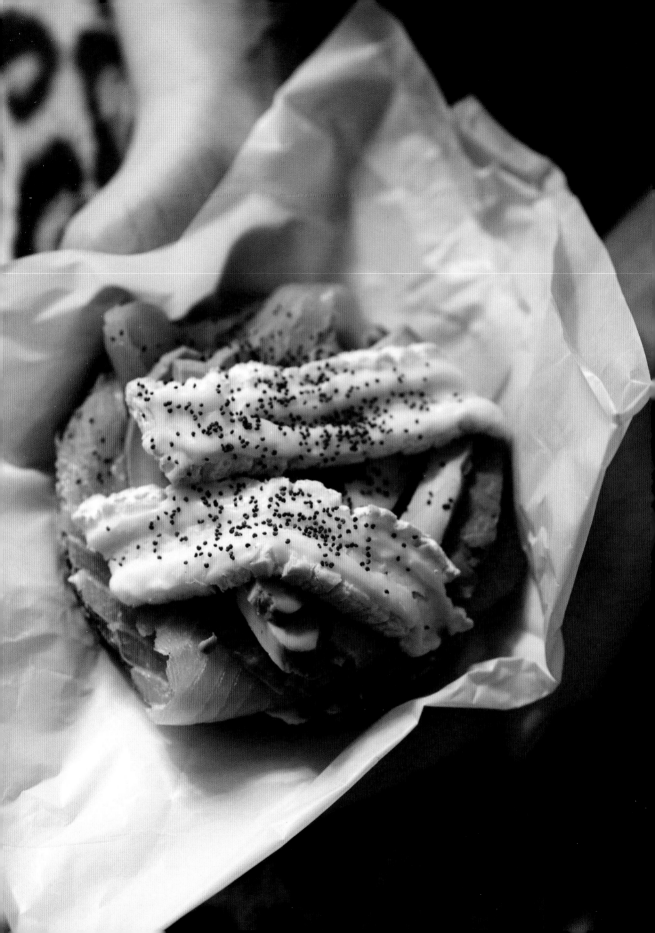

SMOKED SALMON, AVOCADO AND BRIE ON RYE

I'm not really a sandwich kind of a girl as generally I find them too stodgy, but give me bit of brie, some avocado and a little smoked salmon, pop the whole lot on rye and I'm happy. The flavours of the poppy seeds and lemon lift this way out of the ordinary.

1 thin slice of seeded rye bread
(from a small, fresh loaf)
50g smoked salmon
½ small avocado, sliced
a squeeze of lemon juice
30g ripe brie cheese, cut into 2 slices
½ tsp poppy seeds
freshly ground black pepper

Top the bread with the smoked salmon and avocado. Squeeze over a little lemon juice, then lay over the brie. Sprinkle over the poppy seeds and grind over a little black pepper to finish.

383 CALORIES

SERVES 1

PREPARATION TIME

5 MINUTES

CRAYFISH AND GRAVADLAX PUMPERNICKEL

Pumpernickel or rye loaves are both much healthier for you than normal white bread because of their high fibre content. Gravadlax is a cured salmon and can be found by the smoked salmons, while crayfish tails can be found in tubs in good delis or fishmongers.

180g crayfish tails
1 tbsp light mayonnaise
1 tbsp light cream cheese
1 tsp Dijon mustard
zest and juice of 1 lemon,
plus extra for serving
½ a small bunch of dill, finely
chopped, plus extra for serving
sea salt and black pepper
1 beetroot, cooked and finely chopped
4 thin slices of pumpernickel or rye
(from a small, fresh loaf)
4 slices (100g) of gravadlax or
smoked salmon

Drain the crayfish tails if necessary and pop into a small mixing bowl. In a separate small bowl, mix the mayonnaise, cream cheese, mustard, lemon, dill and seasoning. Add to the crayfish along with the beetroot and mix well.

Top the bread slices with the mixture, then lay a slice of gravadlax or smoked salmon over each. Squeeze over a little lemon juice, scatter over a bit more dill and finish with some freshly ground black pepper.

264 CALORIES

SERVES 2

PREPARATION TIME

5 MINUTES

BLACK BEAN TACOS, RADISHES, TOMATOES AND AVOCADO

Healthy tacos? Yup, who'd have thought it? It's important that you get your hands on the really authentic corn tortillas for this. This recipe makes more hummus than you need, but any extra makes a lovely dip with freshly cut crudités – the perfect snack or pre-dinner nibble.

2 small corn tortillas
80g tinned black beans, drained
½ small avocado, chopped
1 vine-ripened tomato, chopped
15g feta cheese, crumbled
a squeeze of lemon juice
sea salt
a small handful of fresh
   coriander leaves
a few dashes of hot sauce, to serve

For the black bean hummus
400g tinned black beans, drained
40g tahini paste
juice of 2 lemons
1 tbsp water
1 tbsp fresh coriander, chopped
1 tbsp extra-virgin olive oil
1 large garlic clove, grated
½ tsp ground cumin
½ tsp ground chilli

To make the black bean hummus, pop all the ingredients into a food processor and whizz until smooth.

Heat the tortillas in a dry frying pan or griddle until lightly toasted. (If you're at the office, pop them in the toaster.)

Spread 2 tablespoons of the hummus across each tortilla. Top with the black beans, avocado, tomato and feta. Squeeze over a little lemon juice and a little sea salt. Scatter over the coriander, shake over the hot sauce and eat immediately.

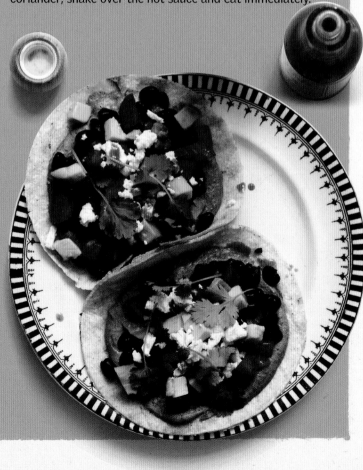

417 CALORIES

PREPARATION TIME **5** MINUTES

SERVES 1

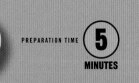 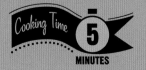
Cooking Time **5** MINUTES

MORTADELLA, PICKLED FENNEL AND ROCKET ON SOURDOUGH

Mortadella is my favourite of all cold cuts. It's garlicky, waxy and, yes, completely processed, but by God is it gorgeous. If you get the chance, try to hunt out the truffle variety – it's possibly the yummiest thing on the planet. The pickled fennel here is easy to make in the evening and is also great as a side with any cold cut or cheese.

---

2 thin slices of sourdough bread
2 tsp olive oil
4 slices (40g) of mortadella
a handful of rocket leaves
a squeeze of lemon juice

For the pickled fennel
1 medium fennel bulb, trimmed,
  cored and very thinly sliced,
  fronds reserved
4 tbsp apple cider vinegar
½ tsp sea salt
¼ tsp sugar
2 tsp extra-virgin olive oil
freshly ground black pepper

To make the pickled fennel, preheat the oven to 200°C/ Gas 6. Place the fennel into a small roasting tray, along with the vinegar, salt, sugar, oil and pepper and rub with your fingers. Roast the fennel for 15 minutes, then turn and roast for a further 10 minutes, until the fennel is golden and cooked through. Leave to cool and set aside until needed.

To assemble the sandwich, heat a griddle pan to smoking, drizzle the oil over the surface of the bread and grill for 3–4 minutes, turning halfway through cooking, until lightly toasted and charred on both sides. Spoon half the fennel onto each slice of toast, then twist and fold 2 slices of mortadella to layer over each. Top with the rocket and squeeze over a little lemon juice. Eat.

210 CALORIES

PREPARATION TIME 5 MINUTES

SERVES 2

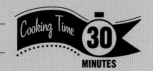 Cooking Time 30 MINUTES

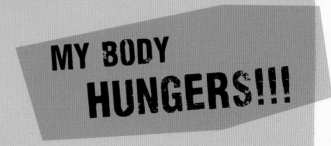

MY BODY HUNGERS!!!

EGGS TONNATO WITH CAPERS, CUCUMBER AND CELERY

When I asked twitter what everyone's favourite sandwich was, most came back saying the simple tuna baguette. I couldn't agree more, so here I've just pimped it, giving it a bit of extra flavour and texture. Tuna purée can be pretty miserable, but done properly it's luscious – creamy and velvety with a lovely, mighty bite. Here it is slathered on top of rye sourdough and studded with soft-boiled quail's eggs, capers, dill, cucumber and celery.

2 quail's eggs
1 thin slice of grainy sourdough bread
1 tsp capers in vinegar
5 thin slices of cucumber
8 thin slices of celery
a few sprigs of dill

For the tuna purée
1 x 200g tin of tuna in brine
2 tbsp 0% fat Greek yoghurt
1 tbsp light mayonnaise
juice of ½ a lemon
sea salt and freshly ground
    black pepper

Soft-boil the quail's eggs in boiling water for 2 ½ minutes. Peel under running water and halve.

To make the tuna purée, put the tuna, yoghurt, mayonnaise and lemon juice in a food processor and blend together to a smooth paste. Season with salt and pepper.

Spread a third of the purée onto the sourdough (the rest can be popped into Tupperware and then put in the fridge, where it will keep for up to 3 days). Scatter over the remaining ingredients. Eat straight away.

240 CALORIES

PREPARATION TIME 5 MINUTES

SERVES 1
(but makes
enough purée
for 3 tartines)

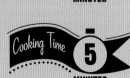 Cooking Time 5 MINUTES

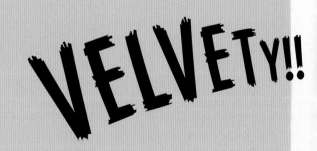 VELVETY!!

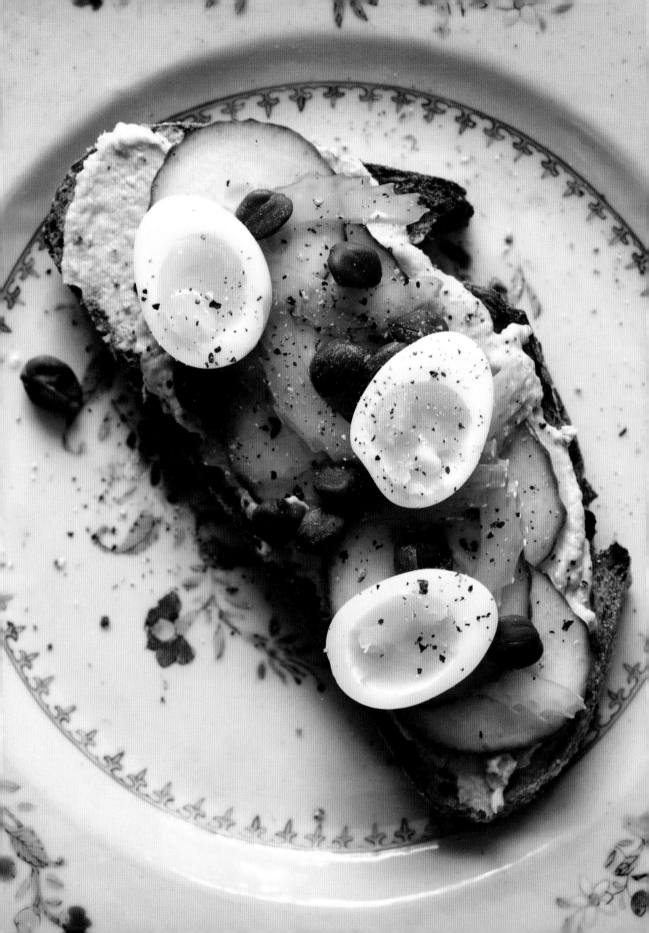

CHICKEN VIETNAMESE BANH MI

The banh mi is a French-Vietnamese baguette filled with paté, salad, mayonnaise, chilli sauce and marinated grilled chicken. This open version is delicious and not too calorie-laden...

1 skinless chicken breast
olive oil spray
¼ baguette
2 tbsp smooth chicken liver paté
2 tbsp light mayonnaise
2 tbsp Vietnamese chilli sauce
8 romaine lettuce leaves, chopped
1 carrot, cut into matchsticks
½ cucumber, peeled, deseeded, and
    sliced into matchsticks
6 spring onions, cut into matchsticks
12 large mint leaves, finely chopped
a small bunch of coriander

for the marinade
1 lemongrass stalk, outer leaves
    removed and very finely chopped
3 lime leaves, thinly sliced
2 garlic cloves, finely chopped
½ tsp turmeric
1 tsp golden caster sugar
2 tbsp fish sauce
1 tsp groundnut oil

for the Vietnamese chilli sauce
2 small garlic cloves, finely chopped
1 small fresh red chilli, deseeded
    and finely chopped
3 tbsp golden caster sugar
juice of ½ lime
100ml rice-wine vinegar
100ml fish sauce
50ml water

To make the marinade, put all the ingredients in a bowl and mix together. Rub the chicken with the mixture then leave to marinate for at least 30 minutes, or ideally overnight.

To make the sauce, combine the garlic, chilli and sugar in a mortar and pound into a fine paste. Add the lime juice, vinegar, fish sauce and water, then stir to blend.

Heat a griddle pan until smoking. Spritz the marinated chicken breast with a little oil, add to the pan and grill for 4–5 minutes on each side, or until golden. Remove from the heat and leave to cool, then cut into slices.

Cut the baguette quarter in half lengthways. To build the banh mi, spread each baguette half with the pâté, then top with the mayonnaise and chilli sauce. Layer over the chicken slices. Toss the lettuce, carrot, cucumber, spring onion, mint and coriander through the sauce and arrange over the chicken. Serve straight away.

GIZZI TIP

This sauce is great for dipping and on salads, so keep whatever you have left over for up to 2 weeks in the fridge.

★ ★ ★ ★ ★ ★ ★ ★ ★ ★ ★ ★ ★ ★ ★ ★ ★ ★ ★ ★

420 CALORIES

PREPARATION TIME **10** MINUTES (plus a minimum 30 minutes marinating time)

SERVES 2

Cooking Time **5** MINUTES

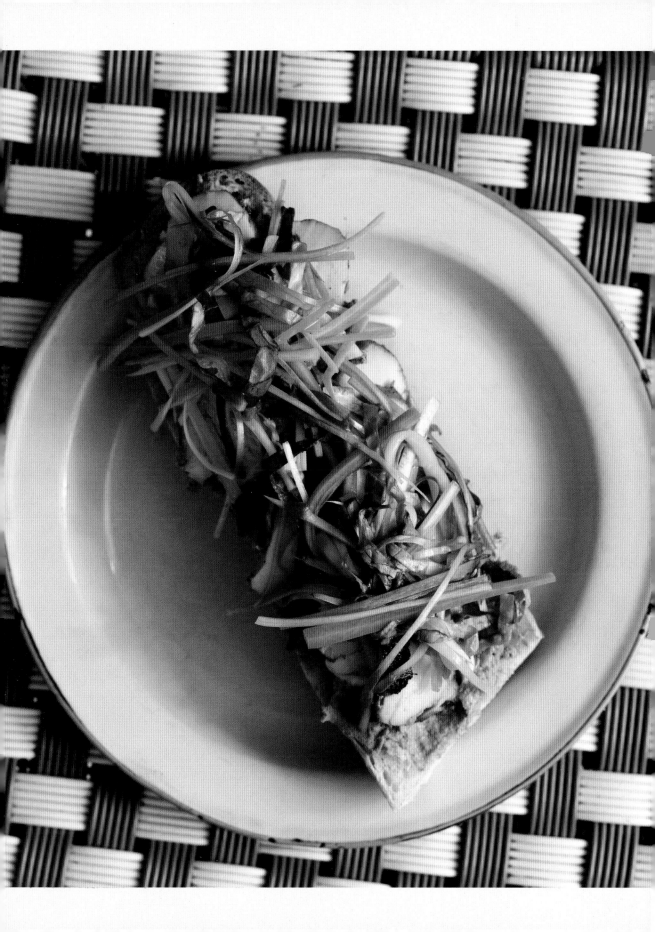

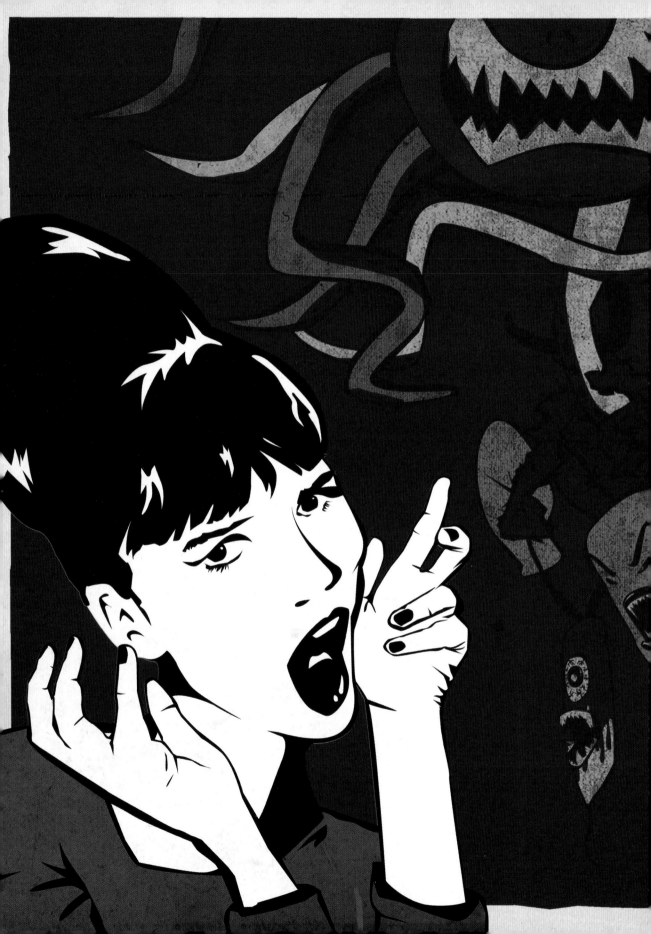

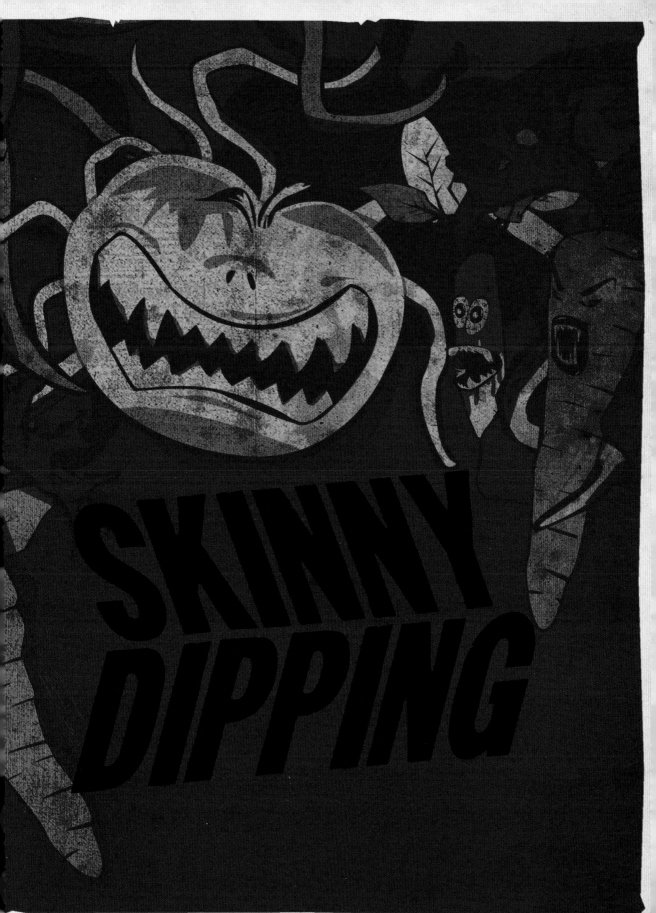

HUMMUS FOR HEROES

I can't remember a time when hummus wasn't in my life. I've been making it since I was at school and my recipe has gone from strength to strength. I used to think that hummus was made up of mostly olive oil, but after studying real Arabic cookbooks I learned that the proper stuff actually uses the cooking brine from the chickpeas to thin it down, with only a spot of oil being used for flavour. This hummus is full of protein and good oils and, though it's quite calorific, it still comes within your daily allowance when eaten with crudités. The toasted pine nuts, pomegranate seeds and mint really do make it a hummus for heroes.

---

for the hummus
1 x 400g can of chickpeas
3 tbsp lemon juice
2 tbsp tahini paste
2 garlic cloves, finely grated
1 tsp sea salt
2 tbsp extra-virgin olive oil

for the topping
1 tsp extra-virgin olive oil
1 tbsp pine nuts, lightly toasted
2 tbsp pomegranate seeds
a few mint leaves, torn
a pinch of cayenne pepper

To make the hummus, drain the chickpeas, setting aside the liquid from the can. Pop in a blender or food processor along with the remaining hummus ingredients, add 50ml of the reserved chickpea liquid and blend for 3–5 minutes on low, until thoroughly mixed and smooth.

Spoon the hummus into a serving bowl and make a shallow well in the centre. Drizzle the olive oil in the well and scatter over the toasted pine nuts, pomegranate seeds and mint. Sprinkle with the cayenne pepper and serve with crudités.

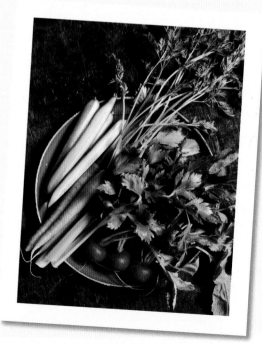

135 CALORIES

PREPARATION TIME **10** MINUTES

MAKES 6
PORTIONS

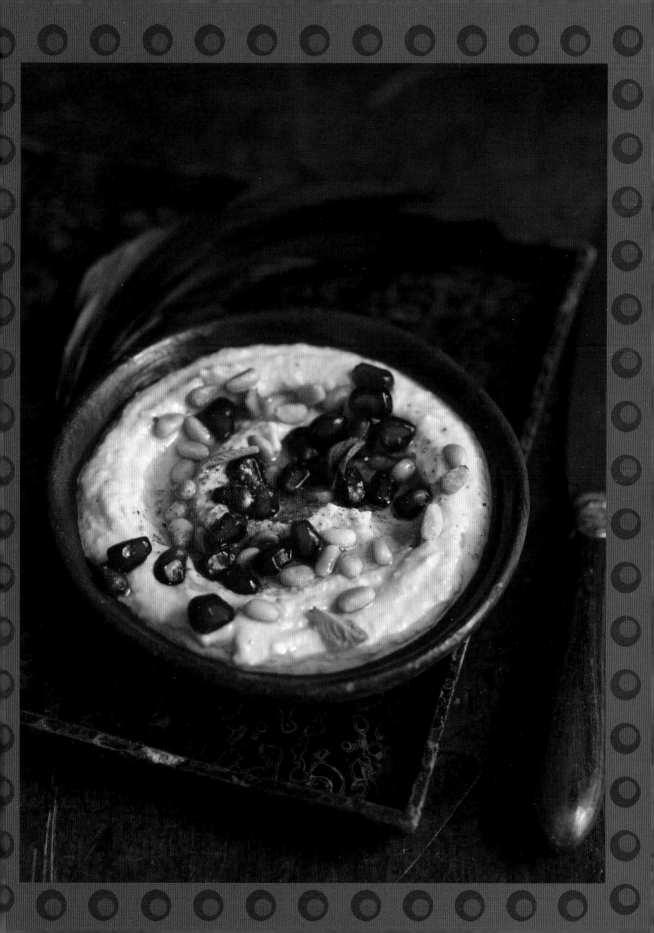

COURGETTE BABA GANOUSH

I've been making baba ganoush for many years before I came up with the idea of making it with courgettes. It's so much fresher and lighter than the aubergine original.

2 large courgettes
olive oil spray
sea salt and freshly ground
   black pepper
1 garlic clove
juice of 1 lemon
1 tbsp tahini paste
100g 0% fat Greek yoghurt
1 tbsp chopped mint

Heat a griddle pan until smoking. Slice the courgettes in half lengthways, spritz with olive oil and season with salt and pepper. Put the courgettes onto the griddle pan and grill for 4 minutes, turning occasionally, until the skin is charred and the flesh has softened. Remove from the heat and leave until cool enough to handle.

Once cool, tip the courgettes onto a board and chop together with the garlic to form a thick pulp. Transfer the mix to a bowl and mash together with a fork to form a thick pulp, then beat in the lemon juice, tahini paste, yoghurt and chopped mint and season with salt and pepper. Serve.

 57 CALORIES

MAKES 4 PORTIONS

PREPARATION TIME **5** MINUTES

Cooking Time **10** MINUTES

SMOKED MACKEREL PATE

I get asked for mackerel pâté recipes more than anything else and it's easy to know why – it's just such a delicious thing, isn't it? I have a wicked recipe which is whipped together with butter and a spot of cream, though it also takes very well to being made low-fat like this.

1 x 100g skinned smoked
   mackerel fillet
a good squeeze of lemon juice
1 tsp finely chopped dill
3 tbsp low-fat fromage frais
freshly ground black pepper

Roughly flake the mackerel into a bowl. Add the lemon juice, dill and fromage frais and beat together with a fork until well combined. Grind over a little pepper and serve.

 85 CALORIES

MAKES 4 PORTIONS

PREPARATION TIME **5** MINUTES

PUREE DE HABAS

I adore this dip, and always order it at my favourite tapas restaurant where it's on the menu. If being wicked it is absolute food heaven with bread dunked in it, though it also takes very well to the plunging of crudités on good days! Though it has a fair bit of olive oil in it, we do need to be getting our oils from somewhere – and olives are one of the best sources.

250g broad beans
1 whole garlic bulb
sea salt and freshly ground
    black pepper
50ml olive oil, plus 1 tsp for drizzling
a sprig of rosemary, leaves stripped
    and chopped

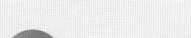

127
CALORIES

PREPARATION TIME **5**

Skin the broad beans, drop into boiling water and cook until tender. Drain and set aside. Preheat the oven to 200°C/Gas 6.

Cut the top off the garlic bulb and season the exposed cloves with salt and pepper. Place on a baking tray, drizzle with a teaspoon of oil and roast for 30 minutes, until the cloves are soft. Leave until cool enough to handle, then squeeze the roasted garlic from the skin.

Pour the oil into a small saucepan over a medium heat, add the roasted garlic and leave to simmer gently for a minute or so. Remove from the heat. Put the broad beans, rosemary and a pinch or two of salt and freshly ground black pepper in a blender, then blitz the ingredients, slowly pouring in the garlicky oil as you do so, to form a silky, fine paste. Return to the pan and heat again until boiling. Serve immediately.

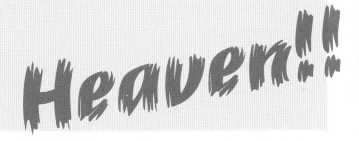

Heaven!!

POPPY SEED TZATZIKI

Tzatziki is a great dip – refreshing and light. The good bacteria in the yoghurt do wonders for digestion, and good digestion means we can metabolise our food better, so it's important we get our fair share of them. This tzatziki has poppy seeds added to it for a bit of extra texture and flavour, as well as upping the protein count.

½ **cucumber,** grated
150g 0% fat Greek yoghurt
½ **green chilli,** deseeded and very
   finely chopped
1 tbsp poppy seeds
sea salt and freshly ground
   black pepper
1 tsp extra-virgin olive oil
a good handful of fresh mint
   leaves, finely chopped

Place the cucumber in a sieve and press down on it with your hands to squeeze out as much moisture as possible. Put the yoghurt in a bowl, add the cucumber, chilli and poppy seeds and season with plenty of salt and pepper. Drizzle over the oil and sprinkle over the mint before serving.

76 CALORIES

MAKES 2
PORTIONS

PREPARATION TIME (10)
MINUTES

GUACAMOLE OF THE GODS

I could eat this by the bucketload. Avocados are full of good fats (hence the high number of calories below) that are wonderful for your skin. For extra crunch and to up this guac's protein and nutritional value, I've served it with toasted pumpkin seeds on top. Not inauthentic, as pumpkin seeds are a massive part of Mexican cuisine.

1 small ripe avocado
juice of ½ lime
a good pinch of sea salt
½ **garlic clove,** grated
½–**1 red chilli,** deseeded and very
   finely chopped
1 tomato, deseeded and chopped
1 spring onion, finely chopped
a pinch of ground cumin
2 tsp pumpkin seeds, toasted

Place the flesh of the avocado into a mortar or a small bowl, and with a pestle or the back of a fork mash the avocado until fairly smooth but still with a few chunks. Squeeze over the lime, sprinkle over the salt and mix together, then add the rest of the ingredients and stir.

136 CALORIES

MAKES 2
PORTIONS

PREPARATION TIME (10)
MINUTES

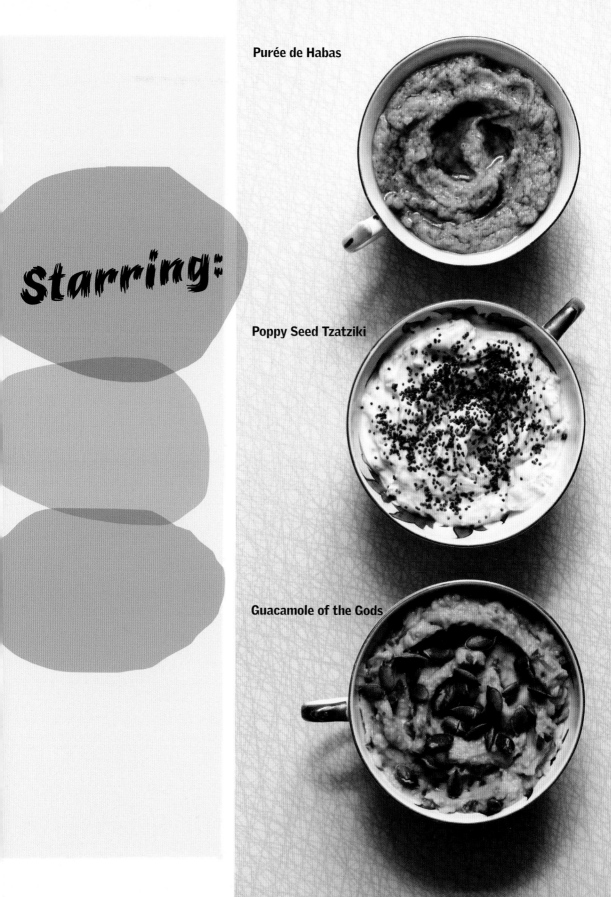

Starring:

Purée de Habas

Poppy Seed Tzatziki

Guacamole of the Gods

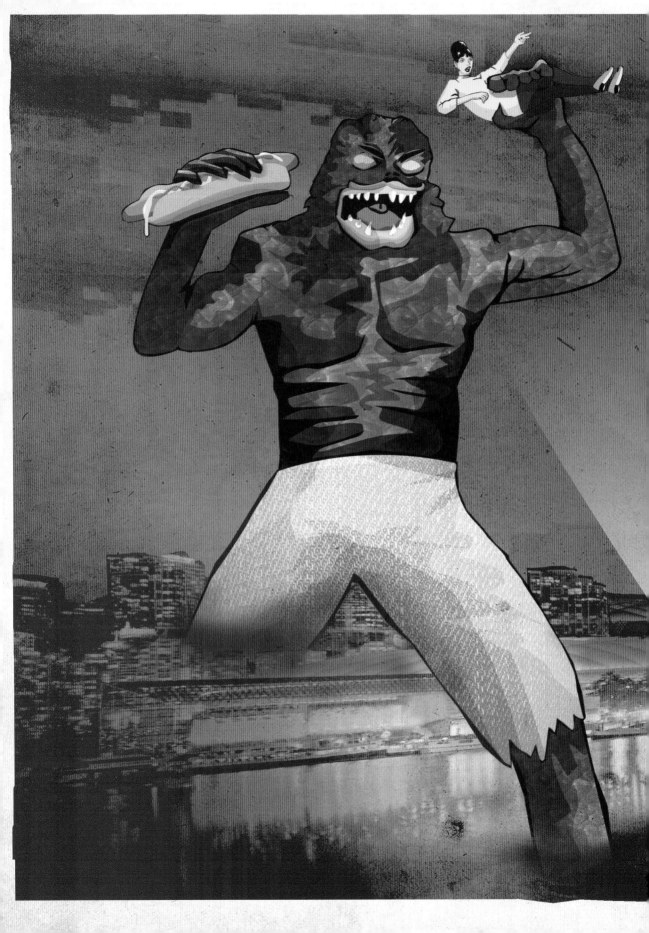

simple
SUPPERS

TUNA TARTARE DONBURI RICE BOWL

Raw tuna is up there as one of my favourite things to eat. I know this may sound scary for an everyday dinner but it's SO easy to make; just make sure you pick up really good sushi-grade tuna from your fishmonger or Japanese supermarket. This recipe is inspired by my favourite Japanese food writer Reiko Hashimoto, whose food is a mixture of authentic and modern Japanese – my kinda cooking. If you are planning on serving it with raw egg yolk, make sure the eggs are very fresh.

200g sashimi-quality tuna
4 tbsp finely sliced spring onion
1 tbsp Japanese Kewpie or
    regular mayonnaise
1 tsp sesame oil
3 tsp soy sauce, plus extra
    for serving
1 tsp wasabi paste, plus extra
    for serving
1 small ripe but firm avocado,
    peeled and chopped into 1cm cubes
120g freshly cooked sushi rice
2 quail's eggs (optional), separated
150g daikon radish,
    cut into matchsticks
1 nori seaweed sheet, shredded

Finely chop half the tuna and roughly chop the remainder (you're after a difference in texture between the two). Put the finely chopped tuna, spring onion, mayonnaise and half the sesame oil in a bowl and mix together gently. Add 1 tsp each of soy sauce and wasabi and mix again.

In another bowl mix together the roughly chopped tuna and half the avocado very gently.

Pop the rice in individual bowls. Arrange the finely chopped tuna mixture around the edge of the bowl, then spoon the roughly chopped tuna and avocado mixture in the centre.

If you are using quail's eggs, make a small well in the centre of each bowl and pop a yolk into each. Scatter over the remaining avocado, radish and shredded nori. Drizzle with the remaining soy sauce and serve with extra wasabi and soy sauce on the side.

PREPARATION TIME **(10)**
MINUTES

SERVES 2

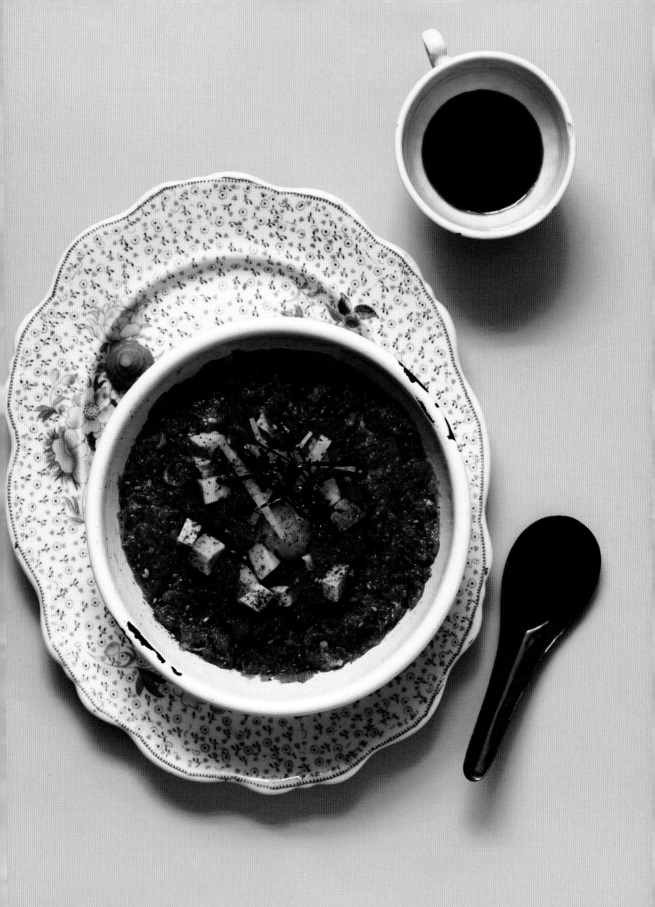

SPICY MISO SALMON UDON NOODLE SOUP

Udon noodles are a thing of beauty. They have a real bite and a silky texture that makes them perfect for slurping. You can use dried ones but I love the fresh ones that you can pick up at Japanese supermakets. Miso soup is perfect for midweek dining – it's so easy to make, it's spicy, it's warming, it's filling and it's virtuous, but most of all, it's absolutely delicious.

---

5 tbsp white miso paste

2 tbsp sugar

2 tbsp mirin

2 tbsp sake

2 x 125g salmon fillets

1 tsp vegetable oil

sea salt and freshly ground black pepper

140g udon noodles

900ml water

1 tsp honey

2 tbsp soy sauce

½ tbsp sriracha (Asian chilli sauce)

6 shitake mushrooms, quartered

50g enoki mushrooms

4 spring onions, green part only, finely chopped

a few chives, snipped into 3 pieces

Put 2 tablespoons of the miso, the sugar, mirin and sake in a small pan and melt gently over a low heat. Leave to cool. Once cool, use to rub the salmon fillets and leave to marinate for 30 minutes to 2 hours.

Heat the oil in a frying pan over a medium heat, then add the salmon to the pan skin-side down and cook for 6 minutes, or until the skin is nice and crisp (be careful not too cook it too fiercely: otherwise the sugar in the marinade will burn). Turn the salmon over and cook for 2 minutes more, or until golden.

Meanwhile, bring a pan of salted water to the boil and cook the noodles according to the packet instructions. Drain and place the noodles in the bottom of two soup bowls.

Add the water, honey, remaining miso, soy sauce, sriracha, mushrooms, spring onions and chives to a pan and bring to just below boiling point. Season to taste, then pour over the noodles, splitting the vegetables between the two bowls. Top with the salmon and serve immediately.

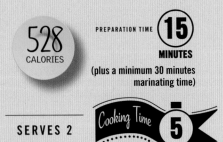

528 CALORIES

PREPARATION TIME **(15)** MINUTES

(plus a minimum 30 minutes marinating time)

SERVES 2

Cooking Time **(5)** MINUTES

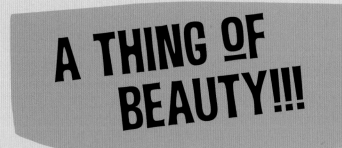

A THING OF BEAUTY!!!

SEA BASS WITH SPROUTING BROCCOLI, CHILLI AND ANCHOVY

I do love fish, and know I should eat more of it, but sometimes I find it's just a bit too pure and not quite buxom enough. Sea bass is a super fish – one of the meatiest around – and it goes well with everything. I adore it like this, though, with the punchiness of the chilli, garlic and anchovy-coated sprouting broccoli.

1 x 500g whole sea bass, cleaned and descaled
sea salt and freshly ground black pepper
olive oil spray
300g sprouting broccoli, trimmed
1 ½ tbsp olive oil
2 garlic cloves, finely chopped
1 red chilli, finely chopped
6 anchovies in oil
1 tbsp chopped parsley

Preheat a grill to high.

Pat the bass dry with kitchen paper, then rub it liberally with salt and pepper and spritz with a little oil. Place the fish on a grill pan layered with foil and pop under the hot grill for 6–8 minutes, or until the skin is crisp and golden. Turn it over and cook for a further 5 minutes on the other side.

Meanwhile, bring a pan of salted water to the boil. Add the broccoli and cook for 2 minutes, then drain. Heat the oil in a wok or frying pan, add the garlic and chilli and cook for 1 minute, stirring as you go so that the garlic doesn't catch and burn. Stir in the anchovies and parsley and cook for another minute, then add the broccoli and coat in the anchovy oil. Serve immediately alongside the fish.

393 CALORIES

PREPARATION TIME **10** MINUTES

SERVES 2

Cooking Time **15** MINUTES

BLACKENED MACKEREL WITH ROASTED TOMATOES AND LIME LEAVES

Mackerel is the Marmite of fish: you either love it or loathe it. I am of the thinking that if you loathe it you probably just haven't had it fresh enough – the problem with oily fish is that they break down and go off pretty swiftly, so you need to get them on the day they hit the your fishmonger's shelves (don't be scared to ask). Mackerel and tomato is a classic combo, but mixed with the zinginess of lime leaves the flavours are lifted to a whole new level.

500g vine-ripened tomatoes
1 garlic bulb, halved
sea salt and freshly ground
    black pepper
1 tbsp olive oil
6 lime leaves, thinly sliced
1 x 400g mackerel, cleaned
    and gutted
1 tsp lime juice

Heat the oven to 180°C/Gas 4 and the grill on high. Wash and dry the tomatoes, then cut in half. Pop them cut-side up into a roasting tray with the garlic, season with salt and pepper and drizzle with half the olive oil. Roast in the oven for 30 minutes, or until the tomatoes have softened and started to char and the garlic is nicely soft. Squeeze the garlic out of its skin and gently stir into the tomato along with the lime leaves. Return to the oven and cook for another 10 minutes.

Meanwhile, grab the mackerel and rub it liberally inside and out with salt, pepper and the remaining olive oil. Place the fish on a grill pan layered with foil, pop under the preheated grill and cook for 6 minutes, or until the skin is crispy golden and charred in places. Repeat on the other side.

When the tomatoes are done, remove from the oven, squeeze over the lime juice and season with salt and pepper. Arrange on a serving tray, placing the mackerel on top. Serve immediately.

422 CALORIES

PREPARATION TIME **10** MINUTES

SERVES 2

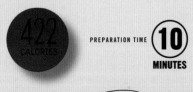 Cooking Time **30** MINUTES

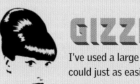 **GIZZI TIP**

I've used a large mackerel for this recipe, but you could just as easily use two smaller fish instead.

★ ★ ★ ★ ★ ★ ★ ★ ★ ★ ★ ★ ★ ★ ★ ★ ★

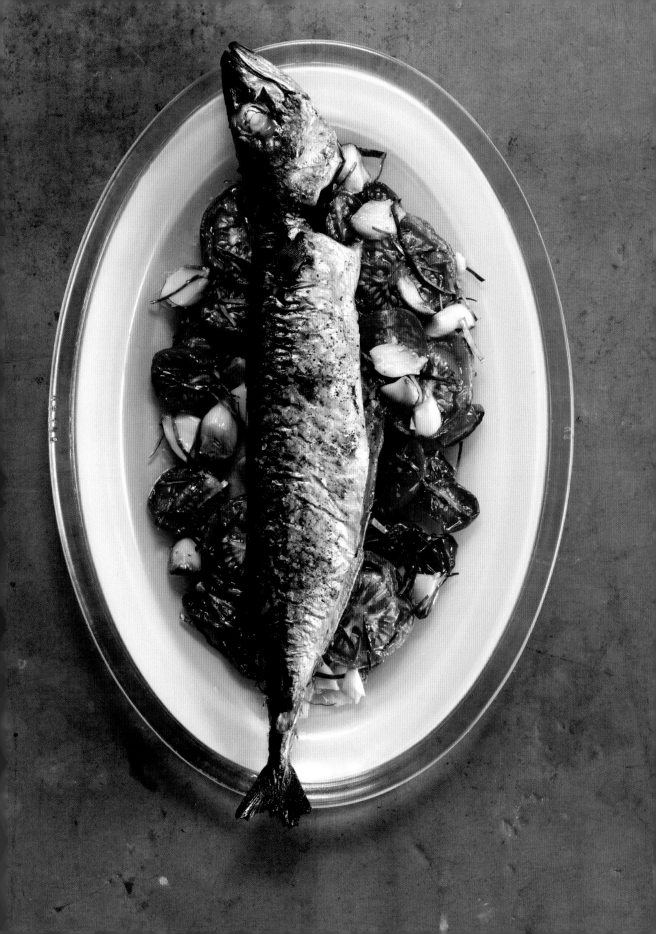

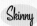

MALAYSIAN FISH STEW

My favourite holiday was in Borneo, where I had this wonderful stew. I love the fusion of different types of cuisine, and the South East Asian, Indian, Chinese, French and Portuguese influences found there made for the most incredible cooking.

---

1 tsp olive oil
1 aubergine, cut into large chunks
2 tbsp tamarind paste
600ml fresh chicken or fish stock
1 tsp palm sugar
1 tomato, cut into wedges
a few springs of mint (Vietnamese
    mint if you can find it)
sea salt and freshly ground
    black pepper
600g red snapper,
    cut into 2.5cm steaks
8 okra
a few mint or coriander leaves
240g cooked brown rice

For the spice paste
1 onion, chopped
6 garlic cloves
a thumb-sized piece of ginger,
    peeled and sliced
10 dried chillies, seeds removed and
    soaked in boiling water to soften
1 red chilli, chopped
1 lemongrass stalk, outer leaves
    removed and finely sliced
1 tbsp toasted shrimp paste
1 tbsp tomato purée
a pinch of sea salt

To make the spice paste, put all of the ingredients into a food processor or blender and blitz until smooth.

Heat the oil in a medium-sized, heavy-bottomed pan. Add the aubergine and fry until golden. Set aside. Add the spice paste to the same pan and gently fry for 3–5 minutes, or until all the liquid has evaporated. Put the tamarind paste, stock, sugar, tomato and mint in the pan, season with salt and pepper and bring to the boil. Lower the heat to a simmer and cook for 15 minutes, or until the sauce is rich and emulsified. Remove and discard the mint, add the fish pieces, okra and aubergine, return to the boil and cook for 5 minutes, or until the fish is just cooked through.

Divide among bowls and scatter over a few mint or coriander leaves. Serve accompanied by 60g of cooked brown rice per person.

PREPARATION TIME **20** MINUTES

SERVES 4

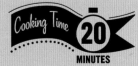
Cooking Time **20** MINUTES

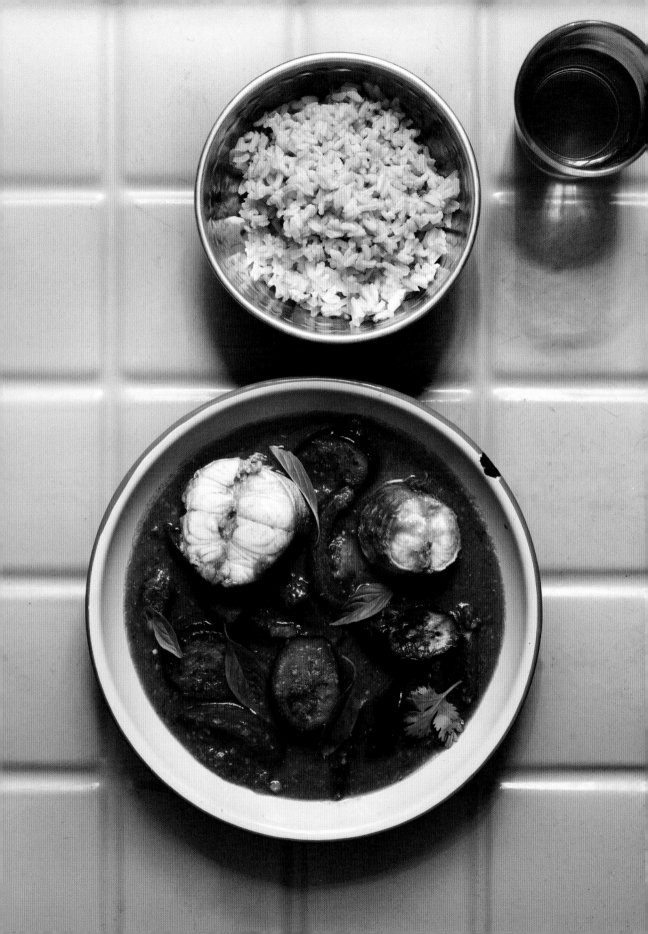

CALIFORNIAN GRILLED PRAWNS WITH GARLIC AND HERB BUTTER AND CHOPPED SALAD

I've been on many a crazy journey since the whole telly thing started, including being lucky enough to have jetted off to LA on a few occasions with work. On my days off when I was able to hang by the pool I would eat this salad for most lunches. Don't be freaked out by the grilled lettuce – the combination of warm salad and hot, garlicky prawns is a winner. Some might be shocked to see butter in the mix of a 'healthy' recipe but the lack of carbs allows us to eat like this. Great, isn't it?

4 gigantic or 6 extra-large prawns, cut in half lengthways and deveined
olive oil spray
sea salt and freshly ground black pepper

For the garlic and herb butter
2 tbsp butter
1 tbsp olive oil
2 garlic cloves, finely grated
1 tsp finely chopped parsley

For the salad
1 head of romaine lettuce, trimmed and halved lengthways
1 ear of corn
1 courgette, quartered lengthways and deseeded
2 vine-ripened tomatoes, chopped
1 small avocado, diced
40ml base salad dressing (page 36)

To make the garlic and herb butter, put the butter, oil and garlic in a pan and heat very gently for about 5 minutes, until the butter has melted and is starting to bubble and the garlic is starting to cook. Remove from the heat and stir in the parsley. Set aside.

For the salad, heat a griddle pan over a medium-high heat. Spritz the lettuce, corn and courgette with oil and season with salt and pepper. Grill the lettuce, turning occasionally, for about 2 minutes or until lightly charred, then coarsely chop it and add it to a large salad bowl. Grill the corn and courgette for a few minutes until lightly charred, then remove the kernels from the corn, chop the courgette and add both to the bowl. Add the tomatoes and avocado to the bowl, pour over the salad dressing and toss to combine.

Pop the prawns in the pan and grill for 2–3 minutes on each side, until golden and cooked through. Divide the salad between plates and top with the prawns. Brush the garlic and herb butter over the prawns and serve at once.

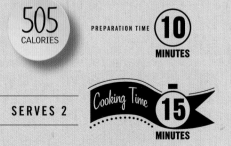

505 CALORIES

PREPARATION TIME **10** MINUTES

SERVES 2

Cooking Time **15** MINUTES

YOGHURT CHICKEN CURRY BOWL

Growing up, my friend Oonagh's mum used to make this dish, and you'd know when she did, as the second you walked through the door the house was filled with the most extraordinary smell. Oonagh's mum's red chicken was marinated and then roasted, tandoori-style, but when making it one lazy day, I cooked the chicken in the marinade and it made the most wonderfully fragrant and bright red curry. It's really good for you, is low in fat and the addition of all the other 'bits' make it a feast for the senses.

500g 0% fat Greek yoghurt
4 tbsp tomato purée
1 large bunch of fresh coriander,
    finely chopped
sea salt and freshly ground
    black pepper
8 skinless chicken thighs, boned
    and chopped into 4 pieces
1 small red onion, finely shredded
1 tomato, deseeded and cut
    into matchsticks
1 mango, peeled, stoned and cut
    into matchsticks
½ small bunch of mint, leaves
    finely shredded
juice of 1 lime
200g cooked brown rice

For the paste
1 tbsp groundnut or vegetable oil
1 onion, peeled and chopped
5 garlic cloves, chopped
a thumb-sized piece of ginger,
    peeled and chopped
2 red chillies, chopped
2 dried red chillies, chopped
1 tbsp ground coriander
1 tbsp ground cumin
½ tsp turmeric
1 tsp paprika

To make the paste, put all the paste ingredients into a food processor and blitz until smooth.

Heat a casserole dish over a low heat, add the paste and toast for 4–5 minutes. Add the yoghurt, tomato purée and half the coriander and season with salt and pepper. Leave to cool fully, then add the chicken thighs and give everything a good stir. Transfer to the fridge and leave to marinate for at least 2 hours, preferably overnight.

Preheat the oven to 180°C/Gas 4. Pop the casserole dish into the oven and cook for 20 minutes, Give it a stir, remove the lid and cook for a further 20 minutes, until the chicken is cooked through and tender and the sauce has thickened.

Put the onion, tomato, mango, mint and lime juice in a bowl and mix together. Divide the rice among 4 bowls and top with the yoghurt curry and onion mix, scattering over the rest of the coriander to finish.

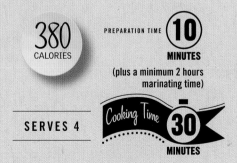

380 CALORIES

PREPARATION TIME **10** MINUTES
(plus a minimum 2 hours marinating time)

SERVES 4

Cooking Time **30** MINUTES

THAI CHICKEN SATAY RICE BOWL

This is a great, fresh take on the classic Thai chicken curry using grilled chicken thighs, yellow curry sauce, peanuts, cucumber, bean sprouts and tons of really fresh Asian herbs. It's blooming delicious and will leave you amazed by how something so familiar can end up being so different. You save about 80 calories if you serve this without the chicken skin, but do cook the meat with the skin attached as it keeps it nice and juicy.

2 chicken thighs, skin on,
bone removed
1 tsp curry powder
a good pinch of sea salt
olive oil spray
30g Thai yellow curry paste
200g half-fat coconut milk
200ml chicken stock
1 tbsp peanut butter
1 tbsp palm sugar
1 tbsp fish sauce
5 lime leaves
120g freshly cooked brown rice
½ small cucumber, deseeded and cut
into matchsticks
4 spring onions, cut into matchsticks
a handful of bean sprouts
1 tbsp chopped toasted peanuts
a small handful each of fresh
coriander and Thai basil leaves

Rub the chicken thighs with the curry powder and salt, then spritz gently with olive oil. Set aside.

To make the sauce, spritz a little oil into the bottom of a pan over a moderate heat. Add the curry paste and fry for 2 minutes. Pour over the coconut milk and chicken stock and add the peanut butter, palm sugar, fish sauce and lime leaves. Bring to the boil, then turn down and leave to simmer for 5 minutes. Keep warm.

Heat a griddle pan until smoking. Lay the chicken thighs into the pan skin-side down, then lower the heat to medium. Grill for 4–5 minutes, until the skin is crisp and lightly charred, then turn over and cook for a further 4–5 minutes, until the chicken is cooked through. Remove from the pan and set aside to rest on a plate for a few minutes. Once rested, cut the thigh meat into thick slices, pouring any excess cooking juices into the curry sauce.

Divide the rice between bowls, then top each with the chicken, sauce, cucumber, spring onions, bean sprouts and peanuts. Scatter over the herbs and serve.

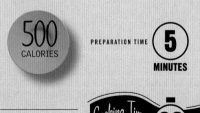

500 CALORIES

PREPARATION TIME **5** MINUTES

SERVES 2

Cooking Time **20** MINUTES

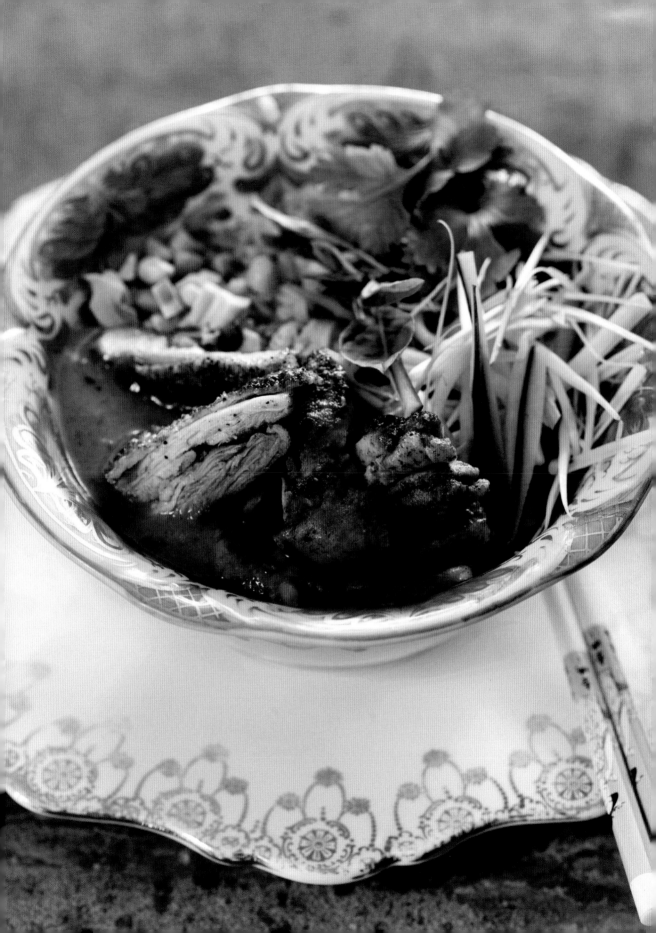

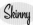

ROAST DUCK NOODLE SOUP

"One duck leg, between two!" I hear your cry. Well, yes, but you'd be surprised by how much meat you get off a duck leg. The soup is also stuffed with other goodies – noodles, greens, mushrooms – you're not going to starve, put it that way! It's a sweet, fragrant and meaty concoction that'll headbutt the winter blues away.

1 x 250g duck leg
sea salt and freshly ground
    black pepper
1 tbsp runny honey
1 tsp Chinese five-spice powder
1 tbsp soy sauce
100g egg noodles
1 litre chicken stock
a thumb-sized piece of
    ginger, sliced
1 garlic clove, bashed
1 star anise
2 tbsp oyster sauce
1 tsp sesame oil
3 shitake mushrooms, quartered
2 heads of pak choi,
    thickly shredded
50g enoki mushrooms
4 spring onions, thinly sliced
a few chives, sliced
1 red Thai bird's-eye chilli, chopped
a few sprigs of fresh mint

Heat the oven to 180°C/Gas 4. Season the duck leg with salt and pepper, lay it on a roasting tray, pop in the oven and roast for 45 minutes, until the skin is crispy and the meat is tender and almost falling off the bone.

Mix together the honey, five-spice powder and half of the soy sauce in a bowl. Heat a saucepan over a medium heat and place the duck leg in the hot pan. Pour over the honey mixture and cook gently until sticky and glossy. Remove the leg from the pan and shred the meat. (Alas, as this is the 'good' part of the week you must – and I apologise for this – get rid of the skin, which harbours most of the fat.)

Cook the noodles in a saucepan of boiling water with a pinch of salt until tender. Drain well.

Heat the stock, ginger, garlic and star anise in a large saucepan, add the oyster sauce, sesame oil and remaining soy sauce and stir to combine. Add salt to taste. Remove and discard the ginger, garlic and star anise from the broth, add the shitakes and cook for 3 minutes, then add the pak choi, enoki mushrooms, spring onions, chives, noodles and duck. Bring to the boil, then remove from the heat. Divide between bowls and garnish with the chopped chilli and mint.

 525 CALORIES

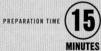 PREPARATION TIME **15** MINUTES

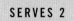 SERVES 2

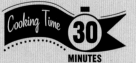 Cooking Time **30** MINUTES

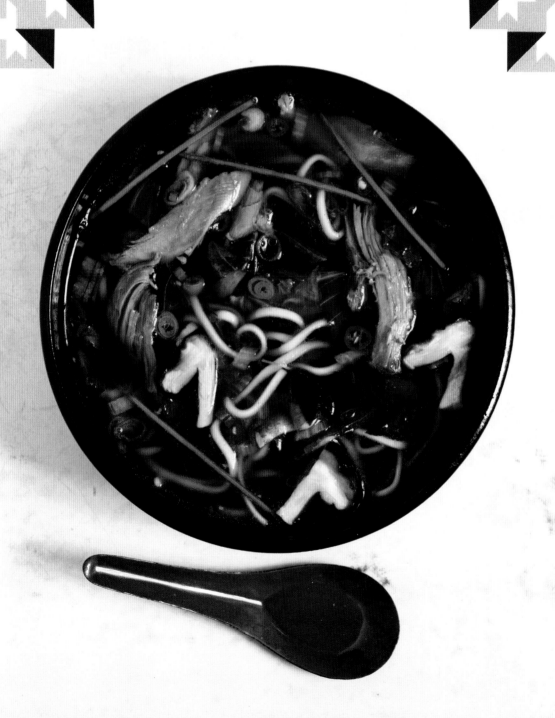

'One duck leg, between two!'

GRIDDLED BABY CHICKEN WITH FATTOUSH, YOGHURT SAUCE AND ROSE HARISSA

In my teens, my sister and I would regularly (and drunkenly) decamp in the dark of night to scoff down shawarma sandwiches in the fantastic Middle Eastern haunts off the Edgeware Road in West London, where we lived. As we grew up, this became more of an event and we would hit the restaurants for really late dinners, spilling in from the clubs, gigs or the theatre to have a proper meal. I would always order the baby chicken and fattoush: always, always, always. As I now live in East London I don't get to do this so often, so I make it myself.

2 x 450g free-range baby
   chickens (poussins)
sea salt and freshly ground
   black pepper
2 garlic cloves, grated
a handful of flat-leaf
   parsley, chopped
1 lemon, cut into wedges, plus the
   juice of 1
1 Lebanese cucumber, deseeded and
sliced into half moons
8 radishes, thinly sliced
½ red onion, thinly sliced
2 tomatoes, chopped
a handful of mint leaves, chopped
1 head of romaine lettuce, shredded
40ml Base Dressing (page 36)
a pinch of allspice
2 pittas, toasted and cut into eighths
½ tbsp sumac

for the yoghurt and harissa sauce
100g 0% fat Greek yoghurt
30g tahini paste
juice of 1 lemon
1 garlic clove, grated
2 tbsp fresh dill, chopped
1 tbsp rose harissa

Put each chicken breast-side up on a chopping board. Insert a sharp, heavy knife inside each and cut right through the centre of the backbone (the one resting on the board). Open the birds flat, then lean on them to make them flatter. Turn them over and carefully remove all the bones from the back with a small knife, then lean on them again to make them as flat as possible. Season the birds on both sides with salt and pepper, then rub with the garlic, parsley and lemon juice and leave for at least 2 hours, or ideally overnight.

Preheat the oven to 190°C/Gas 5 and a large griddle pan to high. Griddle the baby chicken on both sides for 3–4 minutes, or until nicely charred. Transfer to a roasting tray and pop in the oven for a further 8 minutes, or until cooked through.

To make the sauce, mix the yoghurt, tahini, lemon juice, garlic and dill together in a bowl. Dollop the harissa on top.

In a large bowl, combine the cucumber, radishes, onion, tomato, mint and lettuce. Pop the dressing and allspice in a jam jar and shake until emulsified. Pour over the salad and toss to combine. Break the pitta pieces roughly with your hands, add to the bowl and sprinkle with the sumac. Serve the chicken on a plate with the lemon wedges, accompanied by the salad and sauce.

395 CALORIES

SERVES 4

PREPARATION TIME (10) MINUTES
(plus a minimum 2 hours marinating time)

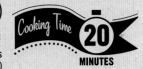

Cooking Time (20) MINUTES

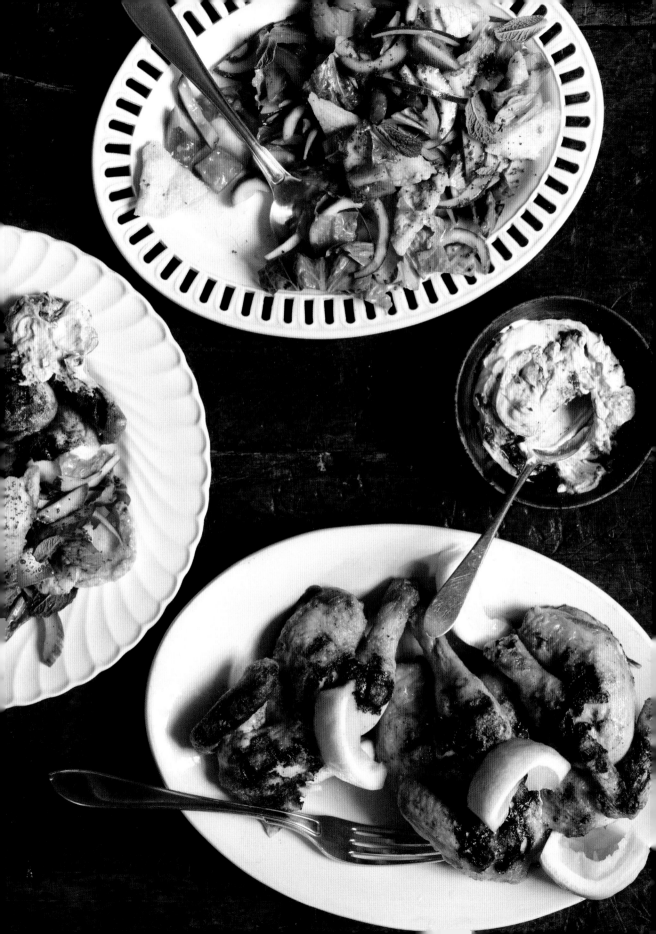

GRILLED MISO TRUFFLE STEAK

I can hear you shrieking, "Truffle, midweek: are you barking?". Truffle oil, though, is such a good reasonable store cupboard ingredient and a little goes a long way. So if you have it in your store cupboard, then why the hell not use it? I make a whopping great portion of this miso sauce – it lasts in the fridge for a good few weeks and is like savoury toffee. It's wonderful slathered on just about everything, but this recipe shows it off on steak. I use onglet as it's a cheaper cut that's also really lean, but if you want to use the more expensive fillet then go wild! And if you still think I'm barking about the truffle oil, then simply omit it. It's still delicious.

50ml sake
50ml mirin
150g white miso paste
50g agave nectar
1 tbsp white truffle oil
1 x 300g onglet steak or
    2 x 150g fillet steaks
200g asparagus spears, trimmed
1 tsp sesame oil
1 tsp sesame seeds (I like a mix of
    black and white)

Bring the sake and mirin to a boil in a medium saucepan over a high heat. Boil for 20 seconds to evaporate the alcohol, then lower the heat, add the miso paste and stir to combine. When the miso has dissolved, return to the boil, add the agave and cook for 1 minute, stirring constantly to ensure it doesn't burn. Remove from the heat and add the truffle oil. Rub your steak(s) with a couple of tablespoons of the miso-truffle sauce and leave to marinate for up to 30 minutes.

Heat a griddle pan until smoking, add the meat and grill for 2 minutes on each side, or until medium rare (I would definitely cook these cuts pink). Whip off the grill and set aside to rest for 5 minutes

Meanwhile, blanch the asparagus for a minute or so in boiling water. Drain, then throw into the pan and grill for a minute on each side. To serve, arrange the asparagus on a plate. Slice the beef and lay it over the top of the asparagus, then spoon 1 tablespoon of the miso-truffle sauce over each steak. Drizzle over the sesame oil and scatter over the sesame seeds to finish.

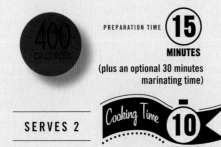

400 CALORIES

PREPARATION TIME **15** MINUTES
(plus an optional 30 minutes marinating time)

SERVES 2

Cooking Time **10** MINUTES

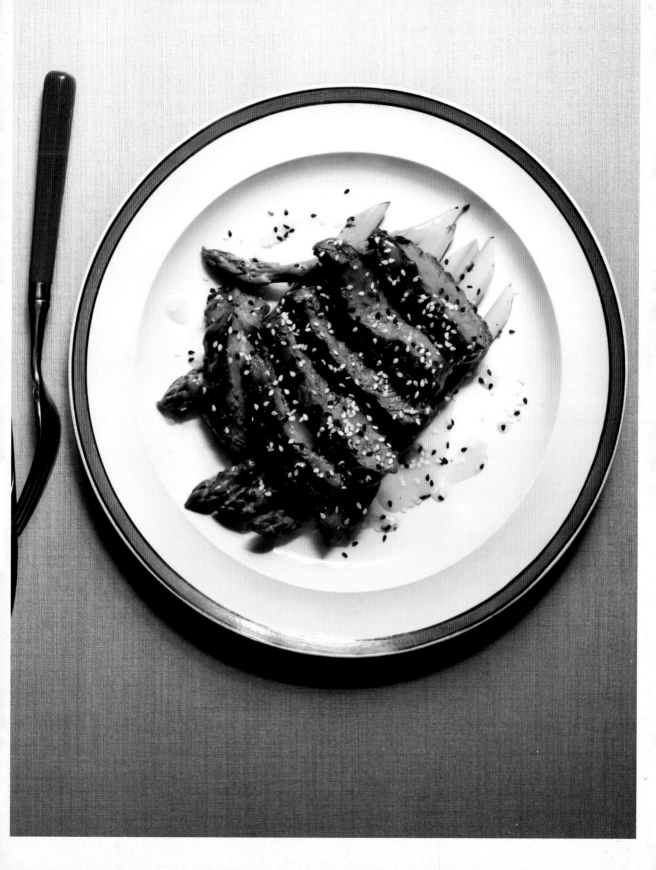

PORK AND CHORIZO MEATBALLS WITH SPAGHETTI

I blooming love meatballs, and these are rather special – the chorizo and chilli pepper give them fire, the fennel lends aroma, and the fresh tomato sauce sets the whole thing off. I'm using spelt spaghetti here; I'm a huge fan of spelt. I find it's easy to digest, and it tastes really good. The spaghetti portion here may seem small, but remember, we eat way too many carbs and I promise you'll still be full after eating this.

200g lean minced pork (10% fat)
150g fresh chorizo sausage, the
   meat extracted from the skin
1 small onion, finely chopped
a few sprigs of oregano,
   leaves removed
sea salt and freshly ground
   black pepper
olive oil spray
320g spelt spaghetti

for the sauce
1 small dried red chilli
½ tsp fennel seeds
4 garlic cloves
2 tsp olive oil
1 small onion, finely chopped
800g vine-ripened tomatoes, halved
1 tsp red-wine vinegar
a pinch of sugar
a handful of fresh basil leaves

570 CALORIES

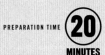
PREPARATION TIME **20 MINUTES**

SERVES 4

Cooking Time **45 MINUTES**

Put the minced pork, chorizo, onion, oregano, and a pinch of salt and pepper in a bowl and mix the lot together with your hands (the chorizo takes a bit of work as it's much firmer than the pork mince). Divide into 12 balls. Pop them on a baking tray, cover with clingfilm and set aside to chill in the fridge.

Meanwhile, make the sauce. Bash the chilli, fennel and garlic together in a pestle and mortar until they break down. Heat the oil in a pan, then add the onions and cook slowly for 8–10 minutes, or until the onions have softened and started to go golden. Add in the crushed garlic, chilli and fennel seeds and fry for 2 minutes. Tip in the tomatoes, add the vinegar and sugar and simmer very gently, uncovered, for about 20 minutes.

Spritz a non-stick frying pan with a little olive oil, then add the meatballs and fry gently over a low heat for 10 minutes, turning them over once. (You may need to do this in batches if your pan is not very big.) Drain off any excess fat, pour in the sauce and cook for a further 15 minutes, then stir through the basil.

Meanwhile, bring a big saucepan of salted water to the boil, add the pasta and cook for 7 minutes, or until al dente. Stir the sauce and meatballs through the pasta and divide equally among bowls.

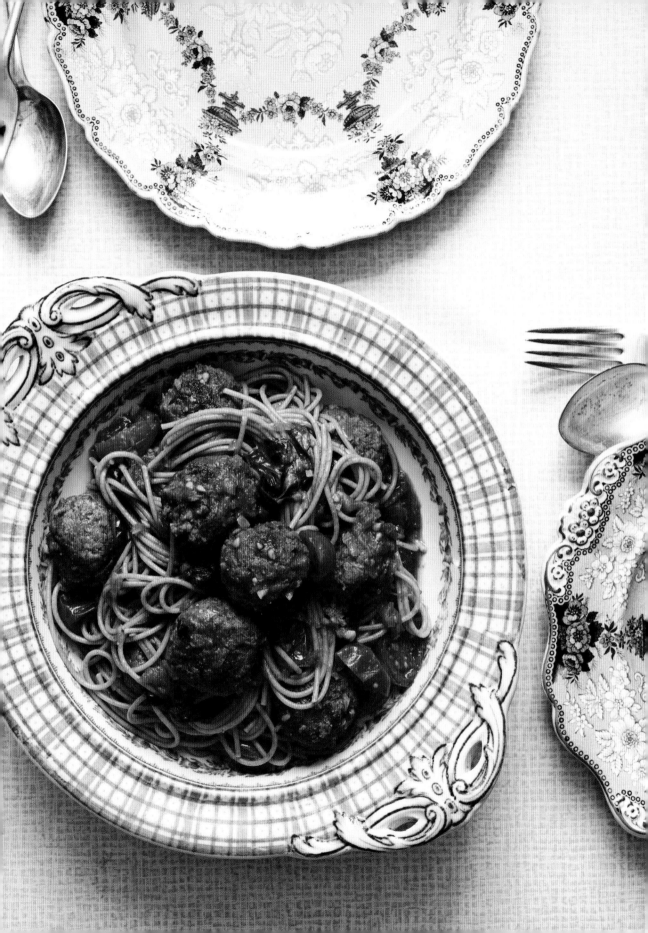

VIETNAMESE PANCAKE WITH PORK, PRAWNS AND TONS OF HERBS

Vietnamese food is fast, fresh and low in fat. It is high in sugar, however, so this and the other Vietnamese recipes in this book are a little less sweet than strictly authentic (though they're still packed with all the right flavours). This pancake is so easy to make and great fun to eat. Just chop it into pieces, wrap it in lettuce with the veggies and herbs and then plunge it into the chilli sauce.

2 tsp groundnut or vegetable oil
200g lean pork mince
200g raw tiger prawns, peeled
    and deveined
1 onion, thinly sliced
1 tbsp oyster sauce
1 tbsp soy sauce
50g bean sprouts
a head of romaine lettuce,
    separated into leaves
a bunch of Thai basil, chopped
a bunch of fresh coriander, chopped
½ cucumber, cut into matchsticks
½ carrot, peeled and cut
    into matchsticks
½ x Nuoc Cham Sauce (see opposite)

for the pancake
50g rice flour
½ tsp ground turmeric
50ml water
¼ tsp salt
50ml half-fat coconut milk
1 tbsp finely sliced spring onion

First, make the pancake. Mix together the rice flour, turmeric and water in a large bowl. Add the salt, coconut milk and spring onion and mix well to form a batter. Set aside.

In a large frying pan, heat 1 tablespoon of the cooking oil over a medium heat until very hot. Add the pork, prawns and onion and stir-fry for 2–3 minutes, then stir through the oyster sauce, soy sauce and bean sprouts. Remove from the heat and spoon out onto a plate.

Return the pan to the heat, adding the remaining tablespoon of oil. Ladle the pancake batter into the pan, tilting to spread evenly, and cook until the pancake is just starting to crisp. Add the pork and prawn mixture to the pan, cover and cook for 2 minutes, until the underside of the pancake is crisp. Fold the pancake in half and cook for a further 2 minutes, until the outside of the pancake is crisp and the inside is soft but cooked. Transfer to a plate.

Chop up the pancake into small pieces and serve alongside the lettuce, herbs, cucumber and carrot. To eat, wrap a piece of the pancake in a lettuce leaf along with the other ingredients and dip into the sauce.

540 CALORIES

SERVES 2

PREPARATION TIME 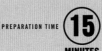 **15** MINUTES

Cooking Time 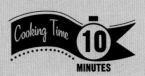 **10** MINUTES

PORK BUN XAO

Bun Xao is a hot and cold salad and is one of my favourite everyday meals. It's made with a base of rice noodles and salad and is topped with grilled or stir-fried meat. It's fresh, fragrant and – with a little of the addictive Vietnamese chilli sauce, nuoc cham, poured over it – spicy.

200g pork fillet, cut into medallions
1 lemongrass stalk, outer leaves
   removed and very finely chopped
3 lime leaves, thinly sliced
2 garlic cloves, finely chopped
½ tsp turmeric
1 tsp golden caster sugar
2 tbsp fish sauce
1 onion, sliced
100g thin rice noodles
8 romaine lettuce leaves, chopped
½ cucumber, peeled, deseeded, and
   thinly sliced into matchsticks
6 spring onions, cut into matchsticks
1 tsp groundnut oil
12 large mint leaves, finely chopped
a small bunch of coriander,
   finely chopped
1 tbsp roasted peanuts,
   finely chopped

for the nuoc cham sauce
1 small garlic clove, finely chopped
½ small fresh red chilli, deseeded
   and finely chopped
1 tbsp golden caster sugar
1 tbsp fresh lime juice
50ml rice-wine vinegar
50ml fish sauce
25ml water

Put the pork medallions on a board and bash them out to form flat discs about 8mm in diameter. Put the lemongrass, lime leaves, garlic, turmeric, sugar and fish sauce in a bowl and mix together. Add the pork and onion to the mixture and leave to marinate for 30 minutes.

To make the sauce, put the garlic, chilli and sugar in a mortar and pound them to a fine paste. Add the lime juice, vinegar, fish sauce and water, then stir to combine.

Put the noodles in a bowl and cover with boiling water. Leave to stand for 10 minutes, or until al dente. Drain under cold water, then divide the noodles between 2 bowls. Mix the lettuce, cucumber and spring onion together and use to top the noodles.

Heat the oil in a griddle pan on high until almost smoking. Remove the pork from the marinade, throw into the pan and grill for a few minutes on each side, or until the meat has charred nicely and is just cooked through. Pop the pork onto a plate to rest for a minute, then slice each medallion into about 4 pieces. While the pork is resting, griddle the onions for a minute or two until nicely charred. Top each bowl with the grilled pork and onions.

Scatter the herbs and peanuts over the bowls and finish with a few tablespoons of the sauce.

466 CALORIES

SERVES 2

PREPARATION TIME **15** MINUTES
(plus 30 minutes marinating time)

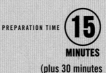

Cooking Time **5** MINUTES

JAPCHAE

I love Korean food – it's very clean, spicy, packs flavour and is really, really light. The glass noodles used here are made from sweet potato, meaning they're low in calories but still give you that satisfying carby feeling. They drink up flavour and are super-fun to eat.

200g dried Korean glass (sweet potato) noodles
2 ½ tsp sesame oil
2 tbsp soy sauce
3 tbsp oyster sauce
1 tsp sugar
1 tbsp vegetable oil
200g lean minced beef (10% fat)
1 onion, thinly sliced
1 carrot, cut into matchsticks
2 garlic cloves, finely minced
a thumb-sized piece of ginger, grated
3 spring onions, snipped into 3
100g shitake or wood ear mushrooms, thinly sliced
150g pak choi or Chinese cabbage, sliced
1 tbsp sesame seeds

Put the noodles in a large pan of boiling water and cook for 5 minutes, until almost cooked through. Drain and rinse with cold water, then toss with 1 tsp of the sesame oil. Use kitchen scissors to cut the noodles into shorter pieces, about 20cm in length. Set aside.

Mix the soy sauce, oyster sauce and sugar together in a bowl.

Heat the vegetable oil in a wok over a high heat, swirling to coat the pan. When the oil is hot but not smoking, add the beef, onion and carrot and fry for about 1 minute, until the vegetables are just softened. Add the garlic, ginger, spring onions and mushrooms and fry for 30 seconds, then add the sauce mix, pak choi and noodles and fry for a further 2–3 minutes, until the noodles are cooked through. Turn off the heat and toss with the sesame seeds and remaining sesame oil. Divide between plates and serve immediately.

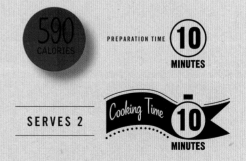

590 CALORIES

PREPARATION TIME **10** MINUTES

SERVES 2

Cooking Time **10** MINUTES

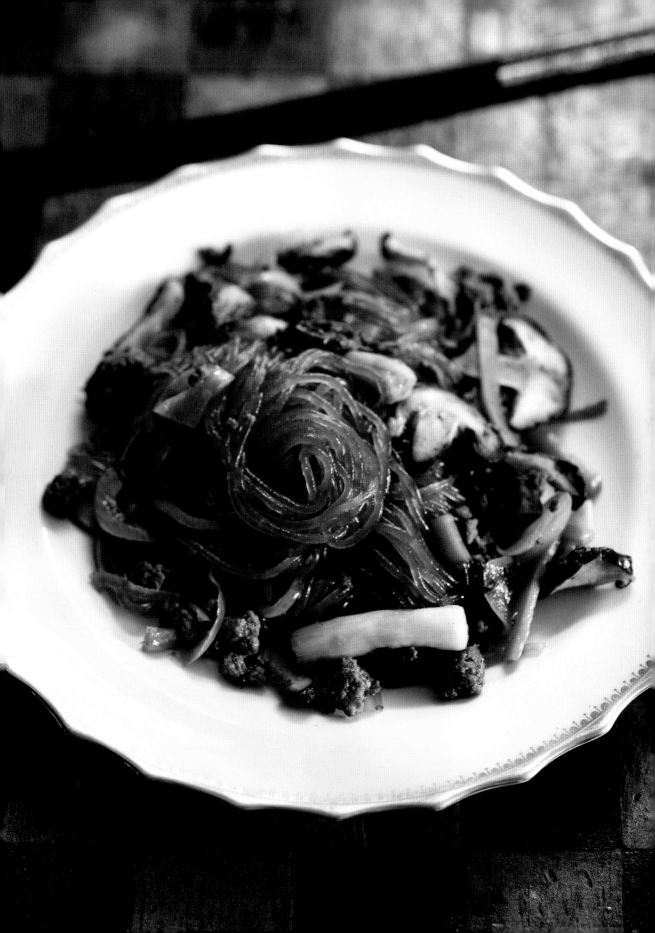

BOLLYWOOD BIRIYANI

All crispy top and gooey sides, this beautiful vegetable biriyani is studded with stunning aromatic toppings. It's an unapologetically gaudy but super-delicious dish.

for the curry
1 tbsp vegetable oil
1 tsp mustard seeds
8–10 curry leaves
1 medium onion, finely chopped
10g ginger, thinly sliced
1 small cinnamon stick
½ tsp turmeric powder
1 tsp each of chilli powder, ground
    cumin and ground coriander
2 green chillies, halved lengthways
2 tomatoes, roughly chopped
1 medium head of cauliflower,
    trimmed and cut into florets
1 x 400g tin of chickpeas, drained
2 tbsp tamarind juice
100ml water
100ml half-fat coconut milk

for the rice
1 tbsp olive oil
2 onions, sliced
10g ginger, grated
¼ tsp turmeric
2 tsp curry powder
a large pinch of saffron
1 star anise
2 cloves
2 green cardamom pods
200g basmati, soaked and drained
2 tbsp 0% fat Greek yoghurt
500ml vegetable stock or water
2 tbsp flaked almonds
the seeds of ½ a pomegranate
1 tbsp rose petals
a handful of coriander leaves

To make the curry, heat the oil in a heavy-bottomed saucepan. Add the mustard seeds and curry leaves and leave to splutter for a few seconds. Add the onion and fry for 10 minutes, until softened. Add the ginger, cinnamon, dry spices and chillies and fry for a further minute. Tip in the tomatoes and cook for 3–4 minutes, stirring well, until the tomato has softened and formed a thick sauce. Add the cauliflower and chickpeas, tamarind juice, water and coconut milk. Bring to the boil, then simmer for 30 minutes, stirring occasionally.

Meanwhile, make the rice. Heat the oil in a deep heavy-bottomed pan over a medium heat, add the onions, ginger, turmeric and curry powder and cook until the onion is tender. Stir in the saffron and whole spices, then tip in the rice and mix together well. Add the yoghurt and stir to coat the rice, then pour in the stock or water.

Cover the pot with a tight-fitting lid, bring to the boil and cook for 2 minutes, then lower the heat and simmer gently for 8–10 minutes. When all the liquid has been absorbed, turn the heat off and leave the pot covered for another 10 minutes. Heat the oven to 200°C/Gas 6. Spoon half the curry onto the base of a clay or cast-iron pot or casserole dish. Top with half the rice then repeat the layers, finishing with the rest of the rice. Scatter over the almonds and bake in the oven with the lid off for 20 minutes.

Serve straight out of the oven scattered with the pomegranate seeds, rose petals and coriander.

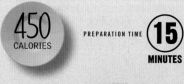

450 CALORIES

PREPARATION TIME **15** MINUTES

SERVES 4

Cooking Time **45** MINUTES

'It will dazzle you with its beauty!'

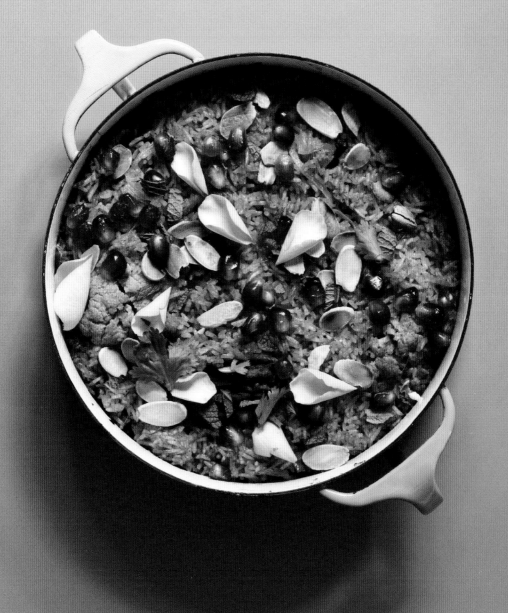

'But its flavours will blow your mind!!!'

PUDS
(if you must...)

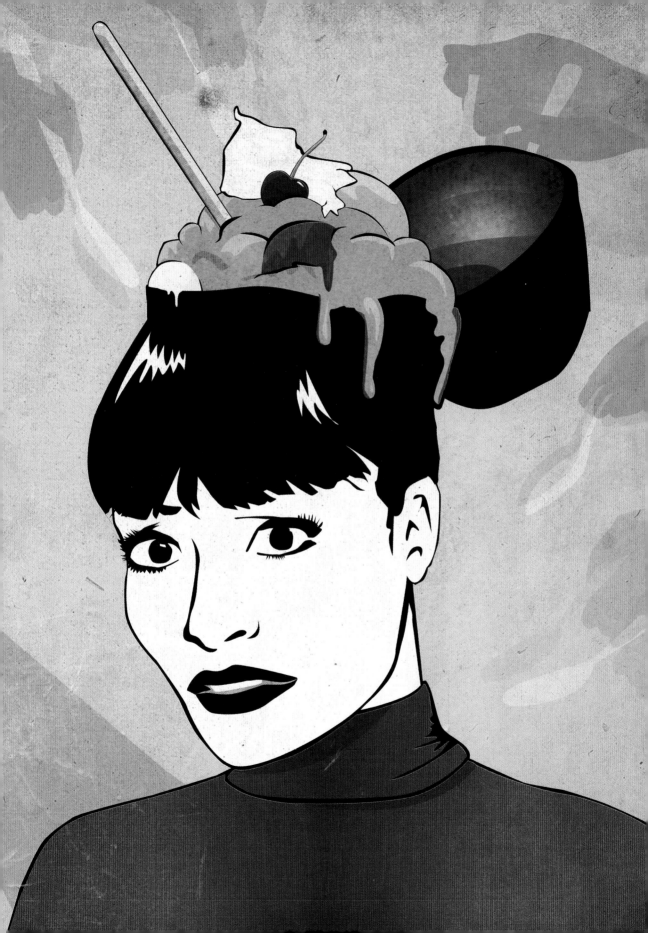

ICED BERRIES WITH HOT WHITE CHOCOLATE SAUCE

Mark Hix created this dish when he was at The Ivy, and in the late '90s you'd find many a supermodel or actress scoffing a portion of it. This was partly down to the minimal calorie content, but also because of its fantastic flavour and the crazy sensation it gives you from eating two foods at such different temperatures.

100g mixed berries (blueberries, raspberries, blackberries, redcurrants, blackcurrants)
15g white chocolate
15ml double cream
1 tbsp Cointreau (optional)

Arrange the mixed berries on a dessert plate, pop in the freezer and freeze for 3 hours, or until solid.

Put the white chocolate and cream together in a bowl over a pan of simmering water and stir continually, until the chocolate has just melted and the sauce is smooth. (Alternatively, pop the bowl in the microwave and cook for a few seconds to melt the chocolate). Stir in the Cointreau.

Take the berries out of the freezer. Drizzle over the white chocolate sauce and serve immediately.

195 CALORIES

PREPARATION TIME **1** MINUTE

FREEZING TIME **3** HOURS

SERVES 1

Cooking Time **5** MINUTES

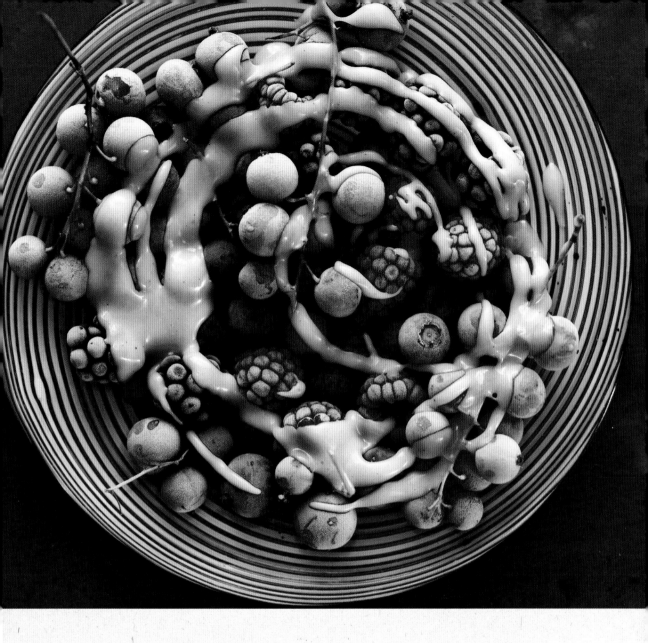

"BBBRRRR!!!"

ROAST BANANA WITH PEANUT BUTTER, MARSHMALLOW AND CHOCOLATE

Utterly filthy good food like this doesn't feel like it belongs in this side of the book, but it does. Though it seems like it's bursting with calories, the naughty ingredients here are only used in tiny quantities, making this a surprisingly low-fat pud.

4 small bananas
2 tsp peanut butter
1 tbsp mini marshmallows
30g good-quality dark chocolate
   chips (70% cocoa solids)

Preheat your oven to 220°C/Gas 7, or its hottest setting. Using a sharp knife, make a cut down the length of each banana and lightly peel back the skin. Spread the peanut butter over the bananas and stuff with the marshmallows and chocolate chips.

Wrap each banana tightly in foil and place on a roasting tray. Pop in the oven and bake for 12 minutes, or until the banana and filling are soft and gooey. Eat immediately.

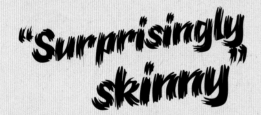

"Surprisingly skinny"

161 CALORIES

PREPARATION TIME **5** MINUTES

SERVES 2

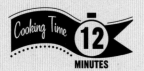

Cooking Time **12** MINUTES

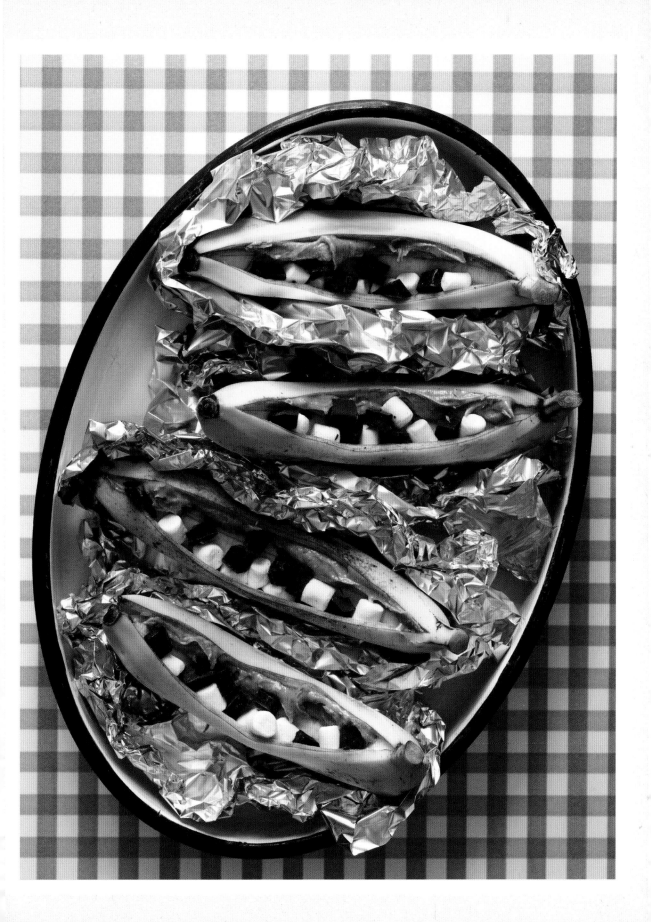

GRILLED PINEAPPLE WITH CHILLI, MINT AND BASIL

This may sound like a pretty weird concoction and, on first bite, I guess it is a little. Soon, though, the sticky sweet pineapple mixes with the chilli, herbs and spices and it becomes clear as to why this is such a great pud.

1 tbsp light muscovado sugar
1 tbsp unsalted butter, softened
1 tbsp dark rum
a handful of mint, finely sliced
10 basil leaves, finely sliced
1 tsp mixed spice
½ medium pineapple, peeled, cored and cut into 2cm discs
a pinch of dried chilli
1 tsp cinnamon

Put the sugar, butter, rum, mint, basil and mixed spice into a small saucepan and stir to combine. Bring to the boil and cook for 1–3 minutes, or until syrupy. Set aside.

Heat a griddle pan until smoking. Using a pastry brush, cover each pineapple disc with a thin layer of the sauce, then sprinkle over the chilli and cinnamon. Add the pineapple to the pan and cook for 4–5 minutes on each side, or until the pineapple rings are slightly charred (you may have to do this in batches, depending on the size of your pan). Serve hot.

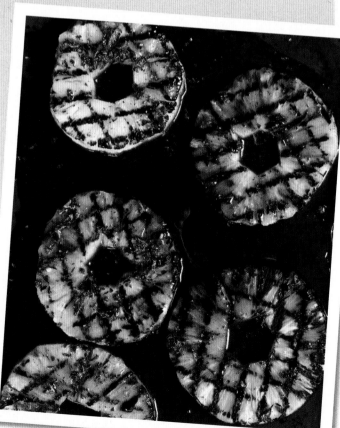

172 CALORIES

PREPARATION TIME **15** MINUTES

SERVES 2

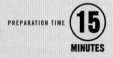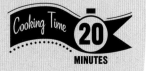
Cooking Time **20** MINUTES

BLOOD ORANGE AND CAMPARI GRANITA

Unlike sorbets, granitas are made with barely any sugar, making them a really good thing to snack on when you find yourself desperate for something sweet. The passion fruit cuts through the sweetness of the blood oranges and the Campari adds a bitter, refined edge.

200ml passion fruit juice (about 10 passion fruits, pulped and sieved)
500ml blood orange juice
100g caster sugar
50ml water
100ml Campari

Put the juices, sugar and water in a saucepan over a low heat. Bring to the boil, lower the heat and simmer for 2 minutes, then remove from the heat. Stir in the Campari and pour into a container. Freeze for 1 hour, then mix the granita with a fork, place back in the freezer and refreeze for 1 hour. Continue this process until the mixture is completely frozen. To serve, scoop one ice-cream scoopful into a glass. Eat straight away.

108 CALORIES

MAKES 8 PORTIONS

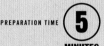

PREPARATION TIME **5** MINUTES

Cooking Time **5** MINUTES

(plus 3 hours freezing time)

AMARETTO SOUR GRANITA

I don't care how naff they are, I could drink Amaretto sours until the cows come home. There's nothing more satisfying than eating this on a warm mid-week evening, knowing you're carrying through with your good intentions while indulging in something wickedly delicious.

200ml lemon juice
80g golden caster sugar
400ml water
100ml Amaretto liqueur
16 maraschino cherries

Put the juice, sugar and water in a saucepan. Bring to the boil, stirring to dissolve the sugar, then reduce the heat and leave to simmer for 2 minutes. Remove from the heat and stir in the Amaretto. Pour into a container and place in the freezer. After 1 hour, remove the granita from the freezer and beat the partially frozen mixture with a fork. Place back in the freezer and refreeze for 1 hour. Continue this process until the mixture is completely frozen. To serve, pop a scoopful of the granita into a glass and top with a couple of maraschino cherries.

99 CALORIES

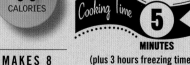

Cooking Time **5** MINUTES

(plus 3 hours freezing time)

MAKES 8 PORTIONS

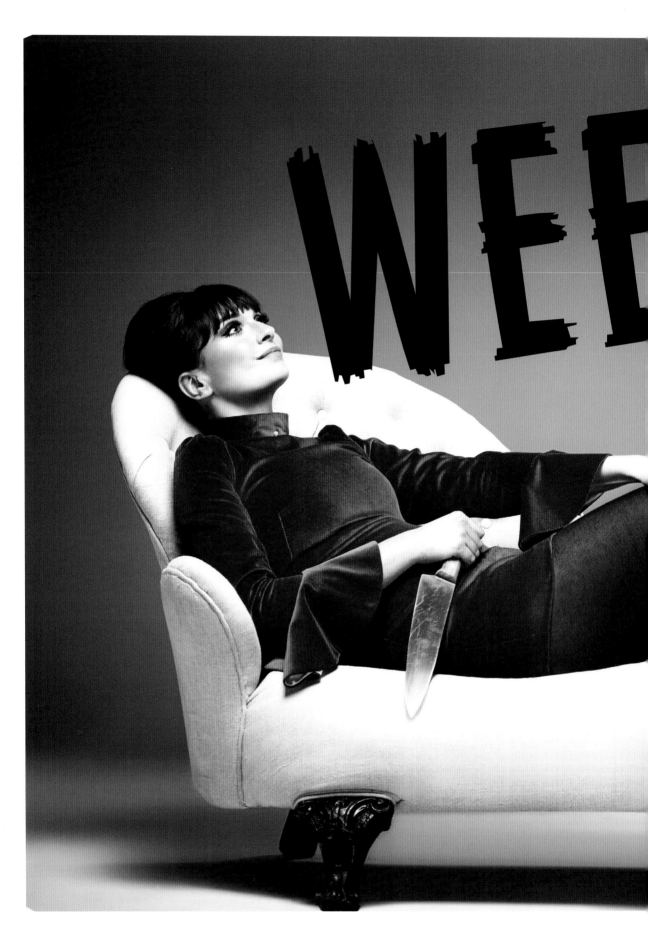

KEND

"FEASTS"

FRIDAY NIGHT FEASTS * LAZY BRUNCHES * SUNDAY LUNCH (AKA THE BIG SHEBANG) * SWEET TREATS

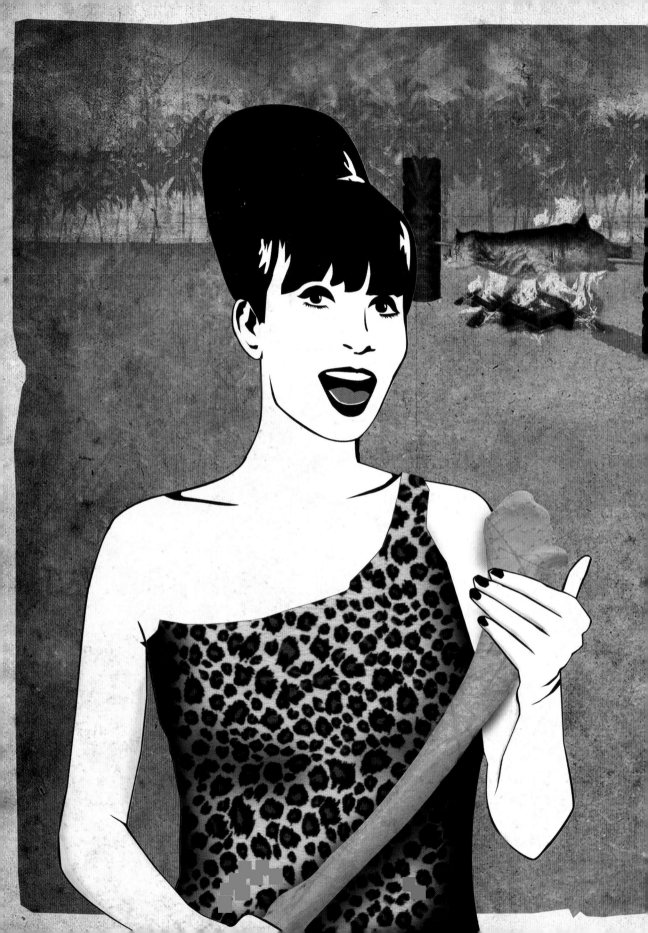

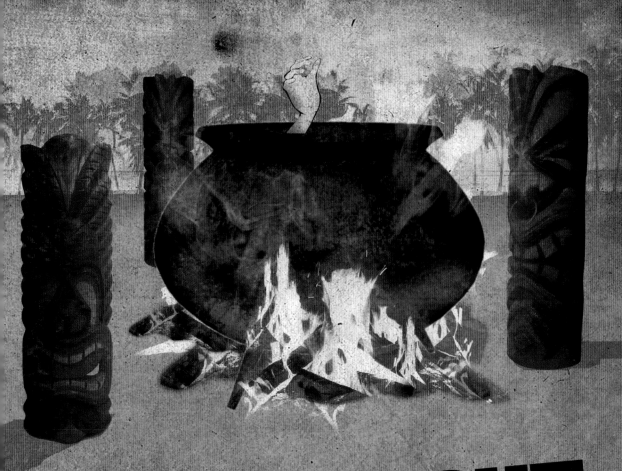

FRIDAY NIGHT
FEASTS

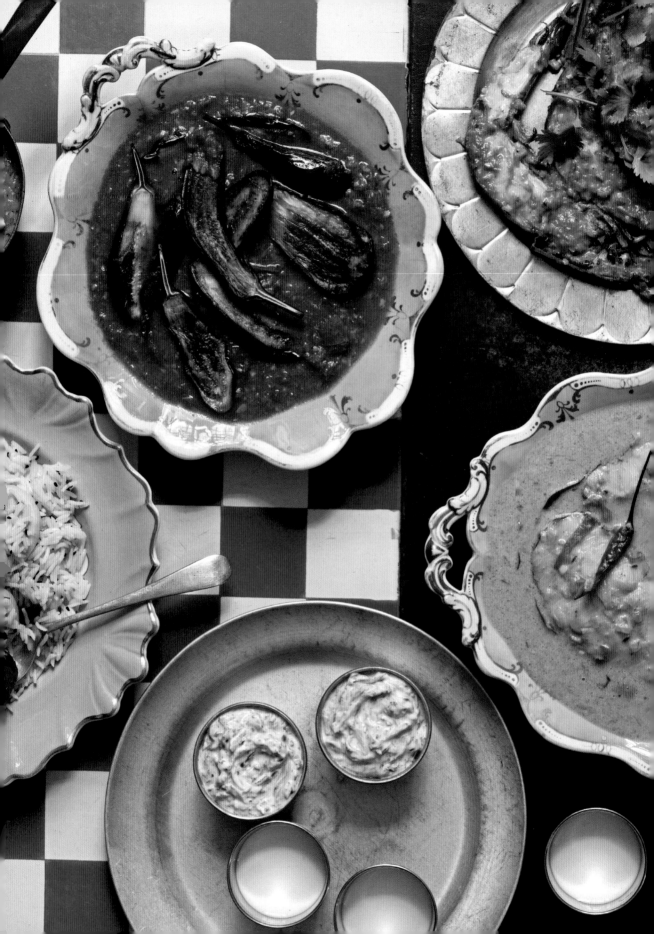

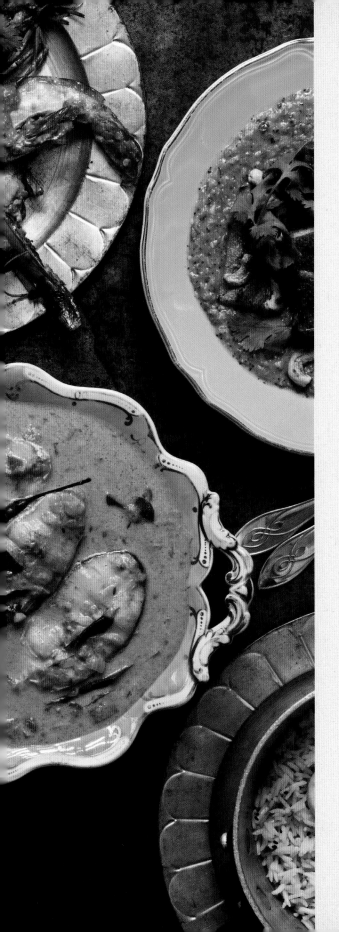

SOUTH INDIAN FEAST

SOUTH INDIAN FISH CURRY
GIANT PRAWNS IN RED CURRY
LEMON RICE
BABY AUBERGINE CURRY
PUMPKIN AND CASHEW NUT CURRY WITH CHILLI RAITA

The southern Indians really are a healthy lot. Their diet is high in coconut, fresh seafood, pulses, aromatics and nuts and seeds, but the thing that sets their cooking apart is the confidence they have in giving vegetables star billing. Here a speedy, fiery, dry prawn curry and a classic lime-perfumed Keralan fish curry are partnered with the sweetness of aubergines and pumpkin, the whole lot served up alongside a surprising spicy raita and a mighty zingy rice. A supper of kings.

SERVES: 6

WICKED RATING 7

Indian FISH Curry

2 tbsp vegetable or sunflower oil
1 tbsp brown mustard seeds
2 tsp cumin seeds
a handful of fresh curry leaves
1 tsp each of garam masala, chilli
    powder and turmeric
3 small green chillies
a thumb-sized piece of ginger,
    grated
6 garlic cloves, finely chopped
1 onion, finely chopped
4 vine-ripened tomatoes,
    roughly chopped
4 kingfish or snapper cutlets
1 x 400ml tin of coconut milk
300ml chicken or fish stock
2 tbsp tamarind juice, made
    fresh from rehydrating
    dried tamarind
sea salt and freshly ground
    black pepper
zest and juice of 1 lime
a handful of fresh coriander,
    roughly chopped

Heat the oil in a large wok, add the dried spices and curry leaves and cook for a few minutes, until the spices release their amazing aromas.

Add the chillies, ginger, garlic and onion and cook for 8 minutes, or until the garlic and onion are soft. Add the tomatoes and a splash of water and cook for a further 5 minutes, then add the fish pieces, coconut milk, stock and tamarind juice and season with salt and pepper. Cover with a lid and leave to simmer for 10 minutes, until the fish is cooked through and the curry has a soupy consistency.

Stir in the lime juice and zest and coriander and serve.

Lemon RICE

Put 240g basmati rice in a pan with 1 sliced lemon, a pinch of saffron, 1 tsp onion seeds and 4 curry leaves. Cover with 1cm of cold water, pop on the lid and bring to the boil. Cook for 5 minutes, or until almost all the water has been absorbed. Remove from the heat and leave to steam for 10 minutes with the lid on before serving.

GIANT PRAWNS in RED CURRY

3 shallots, finely chopped
4 garlic cloves, finely chopped
a thumb-sized piece of ginger,
    chopped
1 red chilli, chopped
2 dried red chillies, chopped
¼ tsp each of ground turmeric,
    cumin and coriander
2 tbsp vegetable oil
4 giant prawns, halved lengthways
    and deveined
a handful of fresh curry leaves
100ml coconut milk
1 tsp brown sugar
1 tbsp tamarind juice

Pop the shallots, garlic, ginger, chillies and spices into a pestle and mortar and pound to a smooth paste.

Heat the oil in a large frying pan until smoking. Lay the prawns cut-side down in the pan and cook for 1 minute until charred. Whip the prawns out of the pan and set aside.

Lower the heat, add the paste to the pan and stir-fry for 1–2 minutes. Add the curry leaves and fry for a further minute, then pour over the coconut milk, sugar and tamarind juice. Pop the prawns shell-side down back in the pan and cook them down in the liquor for about 3 minutes, or until just cooked through, but still opaque in the centres. Arrange the prawns cut-side up on a platter, pour over the sauce and serve.

baby AUBERGINE CURRY

2 tbsp vegetable oil
salt and freshly ground
    black pepper
8 baby aubergines,
    halved lengthways
1 onion, finely chopped
6 garlic cloves, finely chopped
a thumb-sized piece of ginger,
    grated
1 tsp each of chilli powder,
    turmeric and ground coriander
2 tsp ground cumin
600g fresh tomatoes
300g vegetable or chicken stock

Heat the oil in a deep frying pan. Season the aubergines, add to the pan cut-side down and fry for 2 minutes, or until golden. Turn them over and fry for another minute, then remove with a slotted spoon.

Lower the heat, add the onion to the pan and gently fry for 5–8 minutes, or until softened and lightly golden. Add the garlic, ginger and spices and fry for a further 2 minutes, then add the tomatoes and leave to cook down, about 5 minutes. Pour over the stock and simmer for 5 minutes, then return the aubergine to the pan and cook for a further 10 minutes, or until the sauce is rich and the aubergines are cooked through. Season with a pinch of salt and serve.

PUMPKIN & CASHEW NUT CURRY

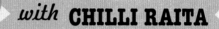

with CHILLI RAITA

600g pumpkin or butternut
    squash, cut into cubes
2 tsp vegetable oil
¼ tsp chilli flakes
¼ tsp cumin seeds
sea salt and freshly ground
    black pepper
1 tbsp each of black mustard,
    cumin, coriander and
    sesame seeds
1 tbsp turmeric
2 onions, chopped
6 garlic cloves, grated
a thumb-sized piece of ginger,
    grated
1 red chilli, finely chopped
100g red lentils
400ml stock
200ml coconut milk
250g cashew nuts, toasted
a handful of coriander leaves

For the raita
3 green chillies
1 garlic clove
a pinch of salt
a small bunch of fresh mint,
    finely chopped
a squeeze of lemon juice
200g 0% fat Greek yoghurt
1 cucumber, deseeded and grated

Preheat the oven to 200ºC/Gas 6. Coat the pumpkin in 1 tablespoon of the oil and rub with the chilli flakes, cumin seeds and a little salt and pepper. Pop on a roasting tray and roast for 20 minutes, or until lightly charred.

Bash the spices and sesame seeds together with a pestle and mortar and heat the remaining oil in a large pan. Add the onions and fry very slowly for about 10 minutes, until they have really softened and started to go golden brown. Add the garlic, ginger and chilli and fry off for 2 minutes, then add the bashed spices and toast them off for 1 minute.

Add the lentils to the pan and stir to coat in the spices. Cover with the stock and coconut milk and bring to the boil, then lower to a simmer and cook for 15–20 minutes. Add the roasted pumpkin and half the cashew nuts and cook for a further 10 minutes, or until the lentils are soft.

To make the raita, add the chillies to a dry pan and gently toast until the skins blacken and blister. Leave until cool, then peel off the skins. Add the chilli, garlic and salt to a pestle and mortar and pound to a paste, then add the mint and lemon juice and pound until the leaves have broken up. Stir this paste into the yoghurt. Put the cucumber in a sieve and press down on it to drain. Pat the cucumber dry with kitchen paper, then stir into the raita.

Serve the curry with the remaining cashew nuts and coriander scattered over, accompanied by the raita.

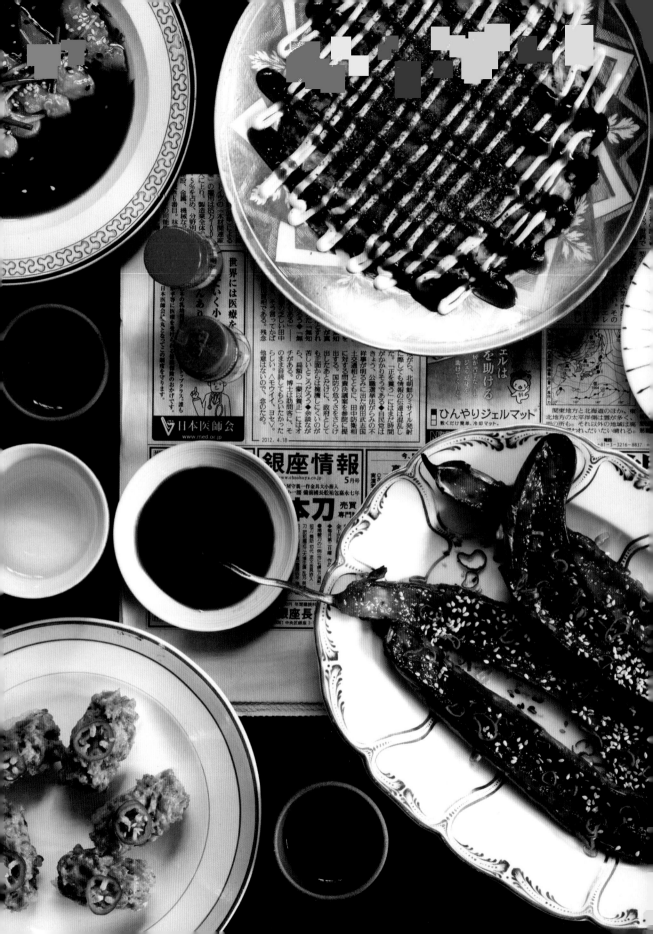

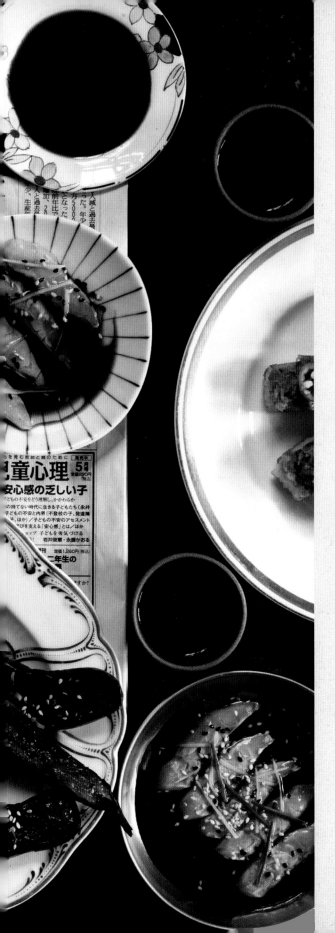

JAPANESE FEAST

CRISPY TUNA RICE
NEW-STYLE SASHIMI
NASU DENGAKU
OKONOMIYAKI

If you're a fan of Japanese food you have to try this feast. Delicious filled Japanese pancakes and flavoursome seared sashimi are accompanied by crisp little sushi rice cakes fried in butter and topped with a spicy tartare – possibly the best thing in the world to eat EVER! If making sushi at home gives you the willies, fear not. I cheat and get my local really good sushi shop to weigh out 12 slices of white fish and simply make the dressing at home to finish the dish off. This way you ensure sashimi-grade freshness, the right cut and you don't have to worry about messing up the slices! Life may never be the same again...

SERVES: 6

WICKED RATING 6

CRISPY TUNA RICE

350g sushi rice
700g water
1 tsp sea salt
2 tbsp golden caster sugar
4 tbsp rice-wine vinegar
250g sashimi-quality tuna loin
1–2 tbsp masago roe
¼ tsp sesame oil
½ tsp sriracha (Asian chilli paste)
2 spring onions, very finely
   chopped
2 tbsp Kewpie Japanese
   mayonnaise
4 tbsp butter
1 green jalapeño pepper,
   finely sliced

Rinse the rice in a sieve until the water runs clear, then add to a medium saucepan with the water and half the salt. Bring to a boil, then reduce to a simmer. Cover and cook for 17 minutes. Remove from the heat and leave to sit for 5 minutes, covered, for the rice to finish cooking in the steam in the pan. Heat the sugar, vinegar and remaining salt over a medium heat until the sugar dissolves, then stir into the cooked rice. Leave to cool.

Hand-chop the tuna as finely as you can. In a mixing bowl, mix the tuna, masago roe, sesame oil, sriracha, spring onions and mayonnaise together. Cover with clingfilm and refrigerate for 1 hour.

Pack large tablespoons of the cooled rice into small block shapes. Flatten each down with oiled hands, so that the rice is tightly packed. Heat the butter in a pan and fry each rice block on all sides for 5–8 minutes, until crisp and golden brown. Place a teaspoon-sized dollop of tuna on top of the rice and finish with a slice of jalapeño.

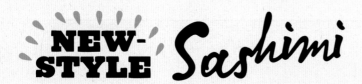

NEW-STYLE Sashimi

120g sashimi-quality sea bass fillet,
   thinly sliced
1 small garlic clove, halved
a thumb-sized piece of ginger,
   peeled and very finely julienned
3 chives, cut into 3cm lengths
2 tsp soy sauce
2 tsp freshly squeezed lemon juice
½ tsp sesame seeds, toasted
1 tbsp extra-virgin olive oil
2 tsp sesame oil

Arrange the fish slices on a plate. Rub the slices lightly with the garlic, then sprinkle over the ginger and chives. Mix together the soy sauce and lemon juice and pour over the fish. Sprinkle over the toasted sesame seeds.

When you're ready to serve, heat the olive and sesame oils in a small saucepan until they begin to smoke. Pour over the fish with a metal spoon – the hot oil will sear the fish as it touches it – and serve immediately.

★NASU ☆ DENGAKU

1 large(ish) purple
    aubergine or 2
    Japanese ones,
    halved lengthways
a drizzle of sesame oil
5 tbsp sweet white miso
1 ½ tbsp mirin
1 ½ tbsp sugar
1 ½ tbsp sake
1 tsp black or white
    sesame seeds
    (or both), toasted

Preheat the grill to medium. Score the cut side of the aubergine(s) in a criss-cross pattern and drizzle over a little sesame oil. Put the miso, mirin, sugar and sake in a small pan and melt together over a low heat. Mix well, then remove from the heat.

Place the aubergine(s) face down on a baking tray and grill for 3 minutes or so. Turn over and grill for a further 5–8 minutes, or until golden and cooked through. Remove from the grill, then spread the miso mix on top of each aubergine half and pop back under the grill for a further minute. Remove, sprinkle with sesame seeds and serve hot.

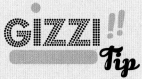

Most of the ingredients for this feast are fairly easy to find, but for the slightly more obscure bits and bobs, take a trip to a Japanese supermarket or check out the Japan Centre online (www.japancentre.com).

OKONOMIYAKI

50g plain flour
75ml dashi or
    chicken stock
1 free-range egg
a pinch of salt
1 tbsp tenkasu (tempura
    flakes), optional
4 spring onions, thinly
    sliced
¼ Chinese cabbage,
    shredded
1 tbsp vegetable oil
2 slices smoked streaky
    bacon, cut in half
    widthways
a good squeeze of
    okonomiyaki sauce
a good squeeze of Kewpie
    Japanese mayonnaise
a shake of togarashi and/
    or sansho pepper

Mix together the flour, dashi or stock, egg and salt in a large mixing bowl to make a pourable batter. Add in the tenkasu if using, spring onions and cabbage and mix to combine.

Heat the oil in a frying pan or pancake pan. Ladle the mixture into the centre of the pan and flatten out with the back of a wooden spoon; you want the pancake to be about 2cm thick and 20cm wide. Round the edges and top with the bacon slices, flattening them into the pancake. Cover the pancake with a lid that fits over the top of it (the lid helps steam the pancake as it cooks) and cook for 3 minutes, or until the base is golden brown

Flip the pancake over, pop the lid back on and cook for another 3 minutes, or until golden and cooked through. Remove from the pan and flip over so that the pancake is bacon-side up.

Squeeze the okonomiyaki sauce over the pancake in horizontal lines, then do the same in vertical lines with the mayonnaise to form a grid. Sprinkle over the pepper and serve piping hot.

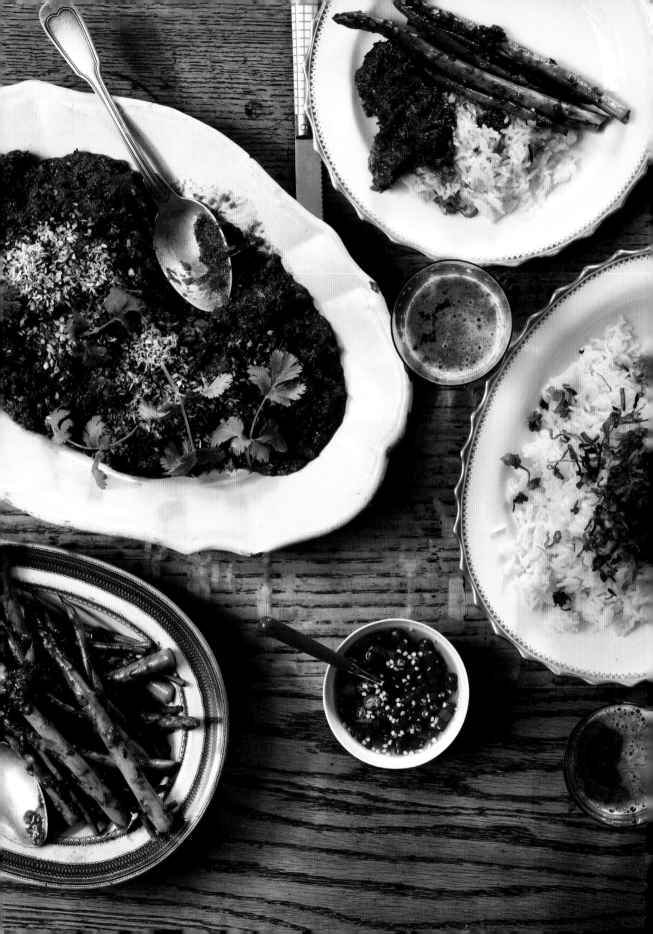

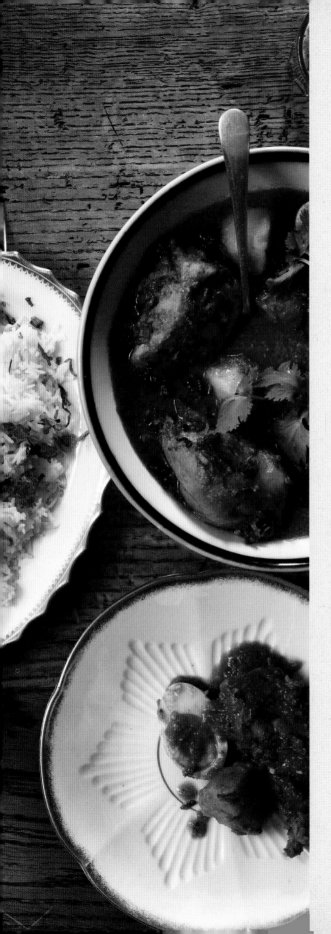

MALAYSIAN
FEAST

**NYONYA CHICKEN
BEEF SHIN RENDANG
ASPARAGUS SAMBAL
FRUIT ROJACK**

I was recently in Borneo and fell head over heels in love with Malaysian food. The mix of South East Asian flavours with the Chinese and Indian influences there makes for a truly delicious, fragrant marriage. Nyonya means 'auntie' in Malay and this is the sort of real family-style cooking I love. This chicken, egg and potato curry garnished with crunchy shallots, hot, sweet and sour chillies and fragrant herbs is always a crowd-pleaser, the slow-cooked beef shin rendang is meltingly good, and the stir-fried asparagus and green beans with sambal is a brilliant way to eat these veg and really showcases this kind of cooking.

SERVES: 6

WICKED RATING 7

NYONYA CHICKEN

with BOILED EGGS, CRISPY SHALLOTS & PICKLED CHILLIES

1 tbsp coconut, groundnut or vegetable oil
1 stick cinnamon
3 cloves
1 star anise
15 curry leaves
1 x 400ml can half-fat coconut milk
200ml chicken stock
1 tbsp fish sauce
2 tbsp palm sugar or light muscovado sugar
1 large organic chicken, cut into 8–12 pieces
500g potatoes, cut into bite-sized pieces
3 tbsp rice-wine vinegar
4–8 Thai red chillies
6 hard-boiled organic eggs, peeled and halved
4 shallots, finely sliced and fried until crisp
a handful of fresh coriander and holy basil

For the paste
4 banana shallots, halved
6 garlic cloves
a thumb-sized piece of ginger, peeled
1 stalk lemongrass, trimmed and chopped
1–2 large dried red chillies, soaked in water for 30 minutes
1 ½ tsp shrimp paste
1 tbsp each of turmeric, ground cumin and ground coriander

Pop all the paste ingredients in a food processor and whiz to a paste.

Heat the oil in a casserole dish, add the cinnamon, cloves, star anise and curry leaves and fry for 30 seconds, or until the curry leaves start to pop. Add the curry paste and toast for 3–5 minutes, until the paste is golden brown.

Pour in the coconut milk, stock, fish sauce and half the sugar, then add the chicken and potatoes to the pan. Bring to a simmer and cook, covered, for 10 minutes. Remove the lid and cook for a further 15 minutes, until the chicken has cooked and the sauce has reduced slightly. (If the breast pieces look as though they are cooked before this time, remove them from the pan, adding them back at the last minute to warm through).

While the curry is cooking, melt together the remaining sugar and vinegar in a small pan. Add the chillies, bring to a simmer and cook for a minute, then remove from the heat and leave to cool.

Add the eggs to the curry a minute before serving to warm through, spoon into a large serving dish and top with the chillies, crispy shallots, coriander and basil.

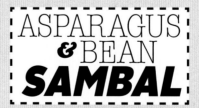

ASPARAGUS & BEAN SAMBAL

Parboil 200g French beans and 200g asparagus until al dente. Drain. Heat 1 tbsp groundnut oil in a small wok, add 2 finely sliced garlic cloves and fry, stirring, for 1–2 minutes. Add the beans and asparagus, 2 tbsp sambal, 1 tbsp soy sauce and 1 tbsp water, stir together until piping hot and serve.

BEEF Shin RENDANG with toasted COCONUT

600g boneless beef shin, cut
    into thick slivers
sea salt and freshly ground
    black pepper
1 tbsp tamarind pulp, soaked
    in 3 tbsp water
1 tbsp coconut, groundnut or
    vegetable oil
1 cinnamon stick
3 cloves
1 star anise
3 cardamom pods
1 lemongrass stalk, bashed
1 x 400ml can coconut milk
2 tbsp fish sauce
200ml beef stock
6 lime leaves, very finely
    sliced
6 tbsp fresh coconut, blitzed
    and toasted, or 6 tbsp
    unsweetened
    desiccated coconut
1 tbsp palm sugar or light
    muscovado sugar

For the paste
5 shallots
    a thumb-sized
    piece of
    galangal,
    peeled
2 lemongrass
    stalks,
    trimmed
    and bashed
5 garlic cloves
10 dried chillies,
    deseeded and
    soaked in warm
    water
2 tbsp water
1 tsp sea salt

Blend the paste ingredients in
a food processor to form a thick
paste. Season the beef with salt and
pepper. Mash and strain the soaked
tamarind, discarding the solids but
reserving the strained liquid.

Heat the oil in a casserole dish,
add the beef in batches and brown
all over. Remove with a slotted
spoon, then add the spice paste,
cinnamon, cloves, star anise and
cardamom to the pan and cook until
they release their aromas.

Return the beef to the pan, add
the lemongrass and cook, stirring,
for 1 minute. Pour over the coconut
milk, tamarind liquid, fish sauce
and stock, cover and simmer over
a medium heat for 1 ½ hours, until
the meat is almost cooked. Stir in
the lime leaves, coconut and sugar,
lower the heat and leave to simmer,
covered, for a further 1 ½ hours, or
until the meat is falling apart and
the gravy has dried up. Serve.

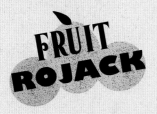

FRUIT ROJACK

600–800g fresh tropical fruits
    (a combination of mango,
    guava, pineapple, star fruit
    and lychees)
1 tsp oil
1 tbsp ground dried
    red chillies
½ tbsp tamarind pulp soaked
    in 3 tbsp water
3 tbsp light muscovado sugar
1 tsp dried shrimp paste
2 tbsp lime juice
100g ground roasted peanuts,
    chopped

Peel the fruit and cut the mango, guava, pineapple and
star fruit into slices (making sure you cut the star fruit
widthways to show its star shape). Pop into a bowl.

Heat the oil in a small pan, add the dried chilli and
toast for 30 seconds. Set aside. Mash and strain the soaked
tamarind, discarding the solids. Reserve the strained liquid.

Combine the tamarind liquid, toasted chilli, sugar,
shrimp paste, lime juice and half the peanuts in a large
salad bowl. Add the sliced fruit and mix well to coat with
the dressing. Divide among 4 plates and top with the rest of
the peanuts. Serve immediately.

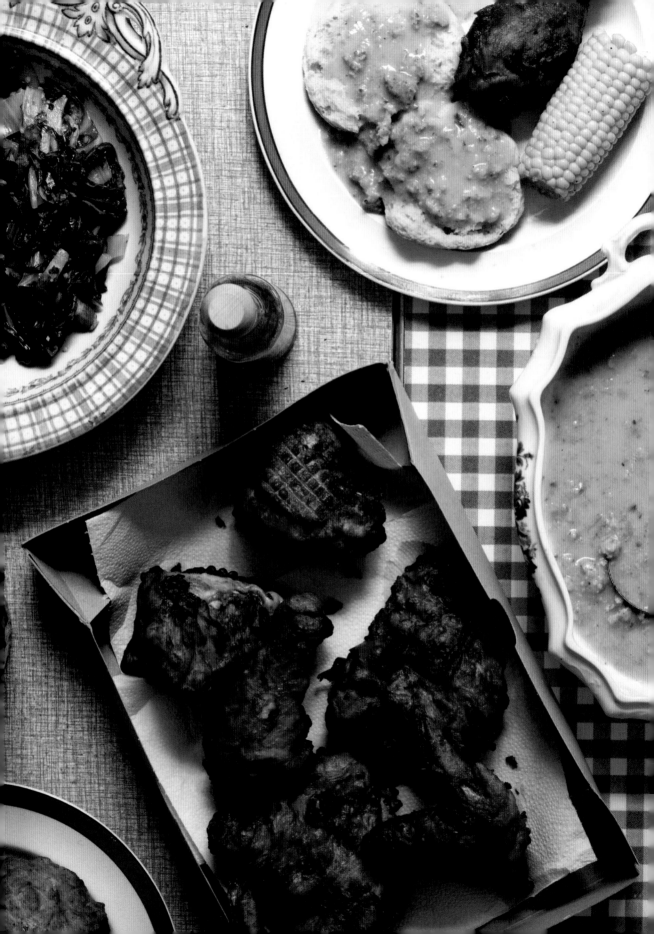

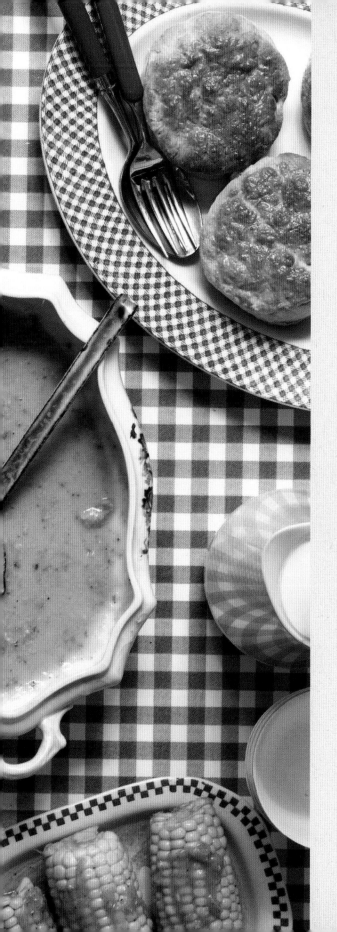

SOUTHERN *fried* CHICKEN FEAST

SOUTHERN FRIED CHICKEN
BUTTERMILK BISCUITS WITH SAUSAGE GRAVY
CORN-ON-THE-COB WITH CHILLI HONEY BUTTER
BRAISED SWISS CHARD WITH BACON

It may not be the most glam of dinners but it's no secret that I'm am obsessed with fried chicken. It's my guilty pleasure. On a recent trip to NYC to feed my obsession, I went to a place called Pies and Thighs, where I had the real deal for the first time ever. I have three words for you. Biscuits. Sausage. Gravy. Suddenly my meal of dreams became EVEN BETTER! So it's the start of the weekend and we're being a bit wicked, (well, in this case very wicked) but if I couldn't eat this once in a while, life wouldn't be worth living! Here's how to do it spectacularly naughtily...

SERVES: 6

WICKED RATING 8

SOUTHERN FRIED CHICKEN

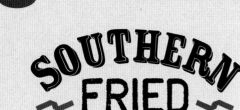

2 free-range eggs
100ml buttermilk
50ml ice-cold water
30–50ml hot sauce
    (depending on how hot you like it)
150g self-raising flour
1 tsp freshly ground black pepper
1 tsp white pepper
1 tsp celery salt
½ tsp sea salt
1 tsp garlic powder
1 medium chicken, cut into 6 pieces
oil, for frying

Beat the eggs and buttermilk together with the water in a bowl, then stir in the hot sauce.

In another bowl, combine the flour and peppers, salts and garlic powder. Dip the chicken in the egg mixture, then coat well in the seasoned flour.

Heat the oil in a deep-fat fryer or wok to 180ºC. Fry the chicken in the oil in batches until brown and crisp, about 8–10 minutes for white meat, 13–14 minutes for dark meat. Drain on kitchen paper and serve immediately.

BRAISED Swiss Chard WITH BACON

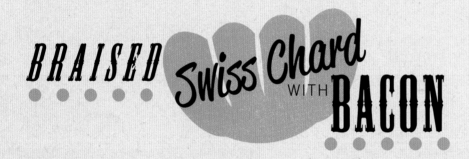

100g smoked bacon or pancetta, cubed
2 cloves garlic, finely chopped
1 red chilli, finely chopped
200g rainbow chard, or plain chard, washed and trimmed
50ml chicken stock

Gently heat the bacon in a frying pan or wok until the fat has begun to render. Increase the heat and fry for 2–3 minutes, then add the garlic and chilli and cook for a further minute, or until the bacon is golden brown.

Add the chard to the pan and fry for a minute, then pour over the stock and leave to braise for 2–5 minutes until tender. Serve alongside the fried chicken.

Buttermilk
BISCUITS
with SAUSAGE GRAVY

1 ½ tsp baking powder
a good pinch of bicarbonate
     of soda
½ tsp sea salt
100g plain flour, plus extra
     for dusting
1 tsp golden caster sugar
1 ½ tbsp ice-cold butter or
     lard, cut into chunks and
     left in the freezer
100ml very cold buttermilk
100ml very cold single cream,
     plus extra for brushing

For the sausage gravy
2 tbsp butter
2 good-quality pork sausages
2 tbsp plain flour
500ml fresh chicken stock
150ml milk
sea salt and freshly ground
     black pepper
¼ tsp white pepper

Heat the oven to 180°C/Gas 4.

In a bowl, whisk together the baking powder, bicarbonate of soda and salt until well combined. Stir in the flour and sugar and mix thoroughly. Rub the butter into the flour with your fingertips, working everything together. Add the buttermilk and cream to the flour mixture and stir together with a wooden spoon to form a dough.

Turn the dough out onto a lightly dusted work surface. Lightly knead the dough, then roll it out to a 3cm thickness. Dust a 5cm cutter with flour, and use it to cut out 8 biscuits. Place the biscuits on a buttered baking sheet, brush with cream or milk and bake for about 12 minutes, or until lightly golden.

Meanwhile, make the gravy. Heat a small wok or frying pan and add the butter. Squeeze the sausage meat from the skins into the pan and fry, breaking it into smaller pieces with a wooden spoon, until nice and golden. Add the flour and cook for 1 minute, stirring, then slowly pour over the stock, stirring as you do so. Stir in the milk and leave to bubble gently for 10 minutes, then season with the salt and peppers.

Pour the gravy into a tureen and pile the warm biscuits onto a platter. Serve the biscuits halved, ladling over the meaty gravy.

CORN ON THE COB
WITH CHILLI HONEY BUTTER!!

Mash together 4 tbsp butter with ½ tsp cayenne pepper, 1 tbsp honey and a little salt and pepper. Transfer to a serving dish.

Bring a pan of salted water to the boil. Cut three ears of corn in half. Plunge the corn into the water and boil for 6–8 minutes, or until the corn is cooked to how you like it. Pop the corn into the dish with the butter and toss until the butter is completely melted and coating the corn. Serve straight away.

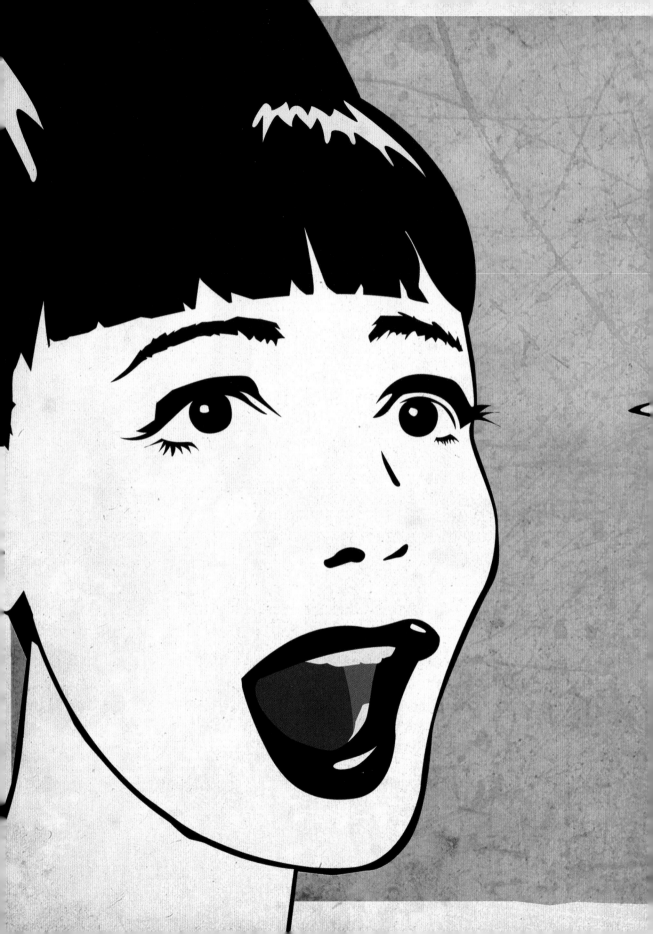

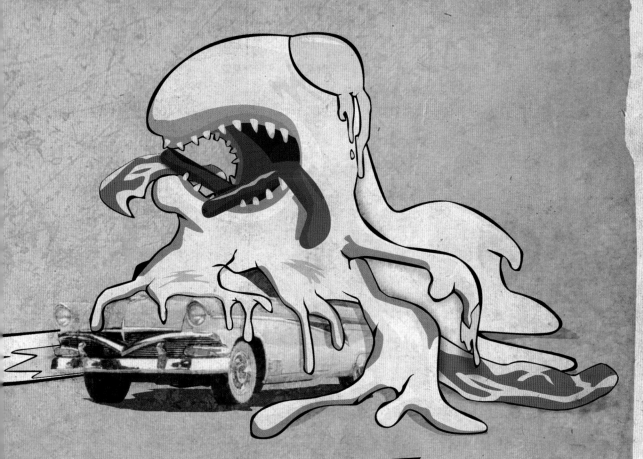

LAZY
BRUNCHES

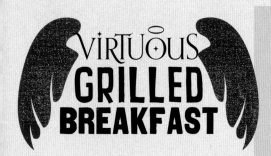

VIRTUOUS GRILLED BREAKFAST

4 portobello mushrooms, sliced
16 cherry tomatoes, on the vine
olive oil spray
2 good-quality pork sausages, skins removed
4 rashers of good-quality lean smoked back bacon, fat trimmed
2 free-range eggs
1 tsp white-wine vinegar
2 slices of sourdough bread, cut on the diagonal
150g blueberries
2 x 250ml glasses of orange juice

I couldn't live without a full English every now and then, but a few little tweaks can make this hangover-beater a lot healthier. Removing the skins from the sausages means that more of the fat they contain is left in the pan, while trimming the fat off the bacon saves hundreds of calories. The mushrooms, tomatoes, blueberries and orange juice help up the fibre content, making the whole thing easier to digest. This may sound a little too healthy considering it's your weekend feast, but this way you get to have the best of both worlds – a bumper English brekky without straying too far from your skinny-week intentions.

Heat the oven to 200°C/Gas 6. Lay the mushrooms and tomatoes on a foil-lined tray. Spray with the oil and roast in the oven for 15 minutes until they have browned and are cooked through.

While the vegetables are cooking, heat the grill to very hot. Shape the sausages into 2 patties. Lay these onto the grill pan and place under the grill for 3–4 minutes, turning occasionally, until cooked. Spray the bacon with oil and grill for 2 minutes on each side.

Meanwhile, fill a small pan three-quarters full of water and bring to the boil. Crack one egg into a cup. Add the vinegar to the pan then, using a wire whisk, swirl the water around to create a whirlpool. Slowly tip the egg into the centre of the whirlpool. When the water comes back to the boil, remove the pan from the heat, cover and leave for 2–3 minutes, then remove the egg with a slotted spoon and drain briefly on kitchen paper. Repeat with the second egg.

Lay the bread on the griddle pan and cook until crisp, about 1 minute each side. Split everything between two plates and serve with the blueberries and orange juice.

SERVES: 2
PREPARATION TIME: 10 MINUTES
COOKING TIME: 15 MINUTES

WICKED RATING 4

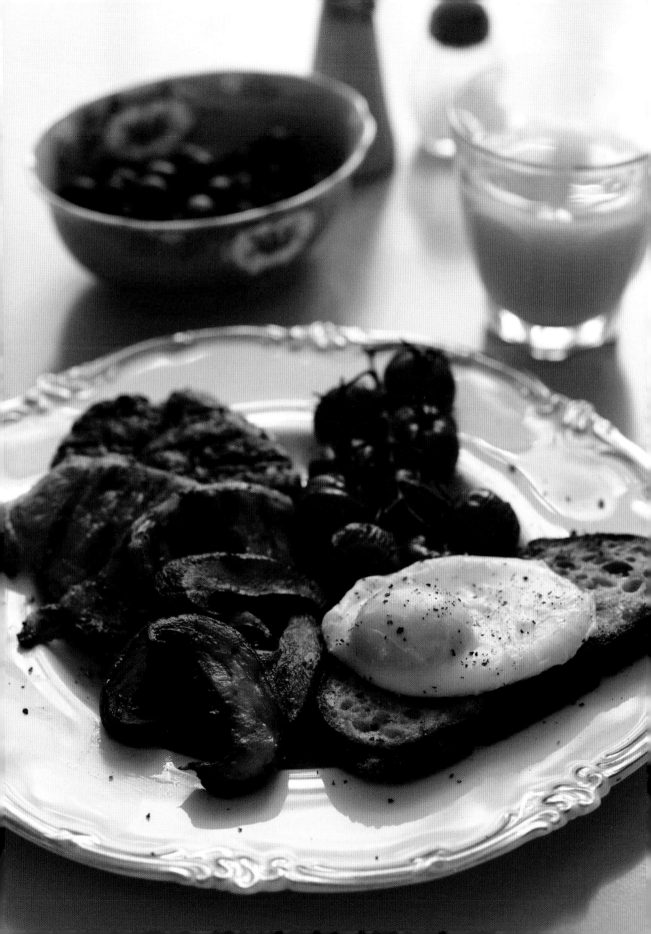

PANCETTA
BAKED BEANS ON TOAST
with
POACHED EGGS

Real baked beans are the bee's knees. My mum used to make them for me growing up and I still can't really stomach the tinned variety as a result. I know it's because I've been spoilt, but I wouldn't want it any other way. Filled with protein and carbohydrates, beans really do give you a spring in your step. Give them a go – they'll leave you running rings round everyone you come across.

1 tsp olive oil
100g pancetta, thinly sliced
1 small onion, chopped
2 garlic cloves, chopped
1 tsp tomato purée
1 tsp red-wine vinegar
1 tsp brown sugar
6 vine-ripened tomatoes, deseeded and chopped
200ml chicken stock
a few of sprigs of thyme
a pinch of dried chilli flakes
sea salt and freshly ground black pepper
2 x 400g can cannellini beans, drained
4 large free-range eggs
4 slices of sourdough bread

Heat the oil in a pan, add the pancetta and gently fry for about 5 minutes, or until crisp and golden. Remove with a slotted spoon and set aside on kitchen paper to drain.

Add the onion to the pan and cook for 5–10 minutes, until the onions are softened and just starting to turn golden. Add the garlic, tomato purée, vinegar and brown sugar to the pan, then stir in the tomatoes, stock, thyme and chilli flakes. Season to taste and simmer for 5 minutes. Add the beans, then simmer for a further 5 minutes, until the sauce has thickened to a silky, coating consistency.

Meanwhile, fill a pan three-quarters full of water and bring to the boil. Crack one of the eggs into a cup. Add vinegar to the pan, then, using a whisk, swirl the water around to create a whirlpool. Tip the egg into the centre of the whirlpool. When the water comes back to the boil, remove the pan from the heat, cover and leave for 2–3 minutes, then remove the egg with a slotted spoon and drain on kitchen paper. Repeat with the remaining eggs. When you've finished all the eggs, pop them back into the water for 30 seconds to reheat.

Heat a griddle pan on high, then griddle the bread on both sides until charred and toasted. Divide the beans, eggs and toast among four plates and serve immediately.

SERVES: 4
PREPARATION TIME: 10 MINUTES
COOKING TIME: 10 MINUTES

 WICKED RATING 5

AUSSIE eggs BENEDICT

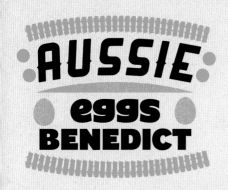

8 large free-range eggs
4 English muffins, halved
 and toasted
8 slices of good-quality
 smoked ham
4 large vine tomatoes, cut into
 4 widthways
2 avocados, sliced

For the hollandaise sauce
2 large free-range egg yolks
½ tsp tarragon or
 white-wine vinegar
a pinch of sea salt
125g cold unsalted butter, cut
 into cubes
a squeeze of lemon juice
a pinch of cayenne pepper

Although I've never been to Australia or New Zealand, I've heard such wonderful things about the food culture over there. The fresh produce and Asian influences seem to encourage some really creative food. They also seem to love an avocado – I've seen loads of recipes where you would never expect to see one! Eggs Benedict is one such example, with many friends of mine coming back from Down Under with tales of the best they'd ever had. Jealous as ever, I decided to take their advice and try my hand at making it this way, which now eclipses the classic for me.

To make the hollandaise, put the egg yolks, tarragon or white-wine vinegar, salt and a splash of ice-cold water in a metal or glass bowl. Whisk continuously for a few minutes, then set the bowl over a pan of barely simmering water and whisk for a further 3–5 minutes, or until pale and thick.

Remove from the heat and slowly whisk in the cubes of butter, bit by bit, until it's all incorporated and you have a creamy hollandaise (if it gets too thick, add a splash of water). Season with the lemon juice and cayenne pepper and keep warm until needed.

Bring a pan of water to the boil. Carefully break an egg into the pan, reduce the heat to a low simmer and poach gently for 3 minutes, or until the white has set around the yolk. Lift the egg out with a slotted spoon and drain on kitchen paper. Repeat with the remaining eggs. (The more confident you get with poaching the more likely you'll be able to poach two eggs at a time). When you've finished all the eggs, pop them back into the water for 30 seconds just to reheat.

To serve, put 2 toasted muffin halves on each plate. Divide the ham, tomato, avocado and eggs among plates and use to top each muffin, then spoon over a generous helping of hollandaise to finish.

SERVES: 4
PREPARATION
TIME: 15 MINUTES
COOKING TIME:
15 MINUTES

WICKED RATING 6

CHORIZO

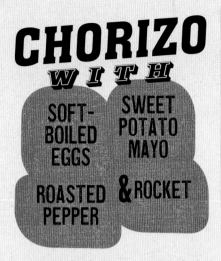

WITH

SOFT-BOILED EGGS

SWEET POTATO MAYO

ROASTED PEPPER

& ROCKET

This could be the ULTIMATE brunch dish – a punchy, flavour-filled way to start the day that will have chorizo fans in their element. There's a little bit to do but, by God, it's worth it. I was introduced to sweet potato mayo by an Australian friend of mine. It's a revelation, and one I'm starting to see pop up on more café menus across London.

1 x 150g(ish) sweet potato
2 tbsp good-quality mayonnaise
4 fresh chorizo sausages, cut in half lengthways
sea salt and freshly ground black pepper
4 free-range eggs
a handful of basil leaves
2 tbsp olive oil, plus extra for drizzling
4 slices of sourdough bread
4 small handfuls of rocket leaves
1 roasted red pepper from a jar, cut into 4 slices

Heat the oven to 180°C/Gas 4. Place the sweet potato on a baking tray and bake for 45 minutes, or until completely soft through. Remove from the oven and leave it to cool completely in its skin. Take the cooked sweet potato flesh from its skin, put in a bowl and mash together with the mayonnaise until combined. Set aside.

Add the chorizo sausages cut-side down to a dry frying pan and fry gently for about 3 minutes, until they just start to get a little charred. Turn them over and cook for a further 3 minutes. Set the chorizo aside and keep warm. (The chorizo will secrete tons of delicious oil while it cooks; save this for later).

Bring a pan of salted water to the boil. Add the eggs and boil for 6 minutes. Remove from the water, drain and peel under cold, running water.

In a pestle and mortar, mash together the basil, olive oil and a little salt and pepper until the basil is completely broken up and the oil is bright green.

Heat a griddle pan until smoking. Drizzle the slices of bread with olive oil, then griddle until toasted and lightly charred on each side.

Spread the toasts with the sweet potato mayo and scatter a handful of rocket leaves over each. Drizzle over a little of the reserved chorizo oil, then top each toast with a slice of pepper and two chorizo halves. Cut the peeled eggs in half and place one on top of each toast. Spoon the basil oil over the toasts and serve.

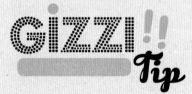

GIZZI!! Tip

To speed up the whole process, I often roast my sweet potato the night before so it's cooled and ready to go by the morning.

**SERVES: 4
PREPARATION TIME: 10 MINUTES
COOKING TIME: 1 HOUR 15 MINUTES**

WICKED RATING 7

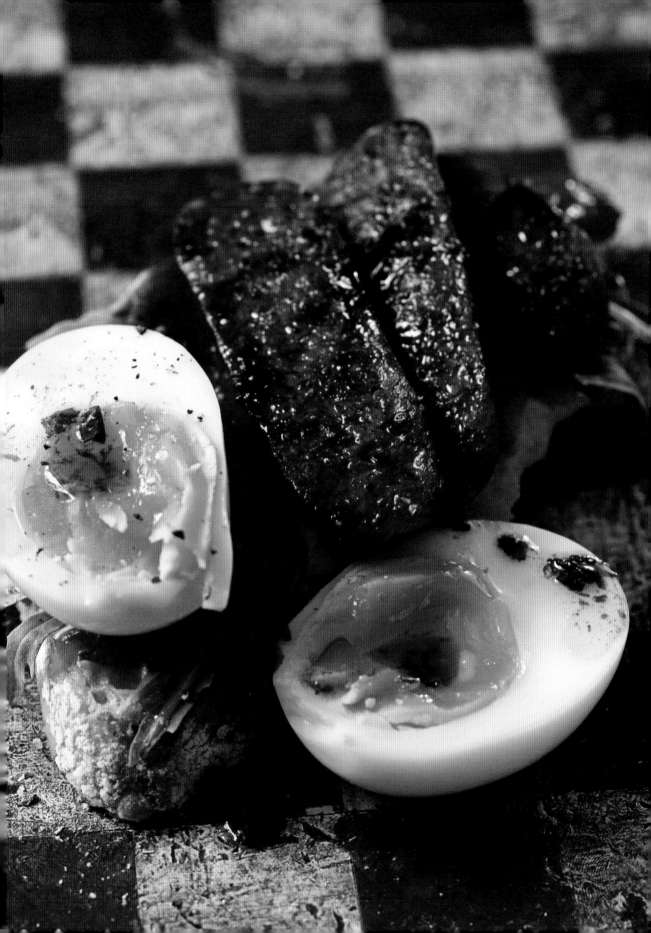

-Quick- CONGEE

with soft Boiled EGGS BROCCOLI CHILLI & Crispy SHALLOTS

Most of Asia embraces congee as the perfect way to start the day, and you'll know why the moment you take your first bite. A savoury rice porridge studded with different toppings, I'm accompanying it with soft-boiled eggs and broccoli here as I think they complement the chilli and oyster sauce perfectly, although you will find that it's not classic. It's also not typically made with rice flakes; however the classic glutinous rice takes forever to cook, while the rice flakes take a good three-quarters off the cooking time.

50g brown rice flakes
600g chicken or vegetable stock
a pinch of salt
a few dashes of soy sauce

For the toppings
1 tbsp vegetable or groundnut oil
2 banana shallots, thinly sliced
sea salt
2 free-range eggs
6 stalks of tenderstem broccoli
1–2 tbsp good-quality oyster sauce
1 red Thai chilli, finely sliced
1 spring onion, thinly sliced

Put the rice flakes, stock and salt in a pan and bring to the boil. Lower the heat to a gentle simmer and cook for 25 minutes, or until the porridge has thickened and the rice is cooked all the way through and pretty much broken up into a mulch.

While the congee is cooking, prepare the toppings. Heat the oil in a frying pan, add the shallots and fry very slowly for about 10–15 minutes, until the shallots are lightly golden and beginning to crisp. Be careful not to burn them. Drain on kitchen paper and set aside.

Bring a pan of salted water to the boil, lower in the eggs and cook for 5–6 minutes. Remove the eggs from the pan, add the broccoli to the water and cook for 1 minute, then drain. Quickly peel the eggs under cold running water and cut them in half lengthways.

Stir the soy sauce into the congee and divide between two bowls. Top each with two egg halves and three broccoli stalks, then shake over the oyster sauce and scatter over the chilli, spring onion and crispy shallots.

GIZZI!! Tip

If you're vegetarian, replace the oyster sauce with hoisin or soy sauce instead.

SERVES: 2
PREPARATION TIME: 10 MINUTES
COOKING TIME: 25 MINUTES

WICKED RATING 5

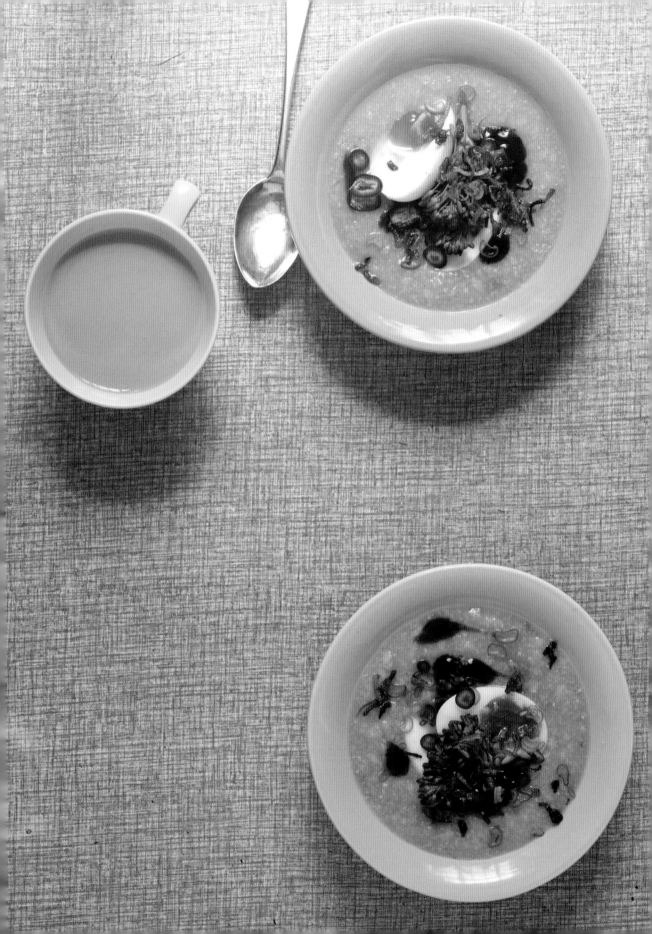

HUEVOS RANCHEROS

I first came across this when travelling round Mexico in my early twenties, and now I don't think a weekend goes by when I don't make it. If anyone stays over after a party this is pretty much always what I cook for them – the chilli and eggs being the perfect antidote to a night's boozing. Truly the best way to ease yourself into a hungover Sunday...

1 tbsp olive oil
4 garlic cloves, finely chopped
1 red chilli, finely chopped
1 x 400g tin chopped tomatoes
1 tbsp tomato purée
a splash of red-wine vinegar
a good handful of fresh
    coriander, chopped
sea salt and freshly ground
    black pepper
1 x 200g can refried beans
    (optional)
4 small corn tortillas
2–3 tbsp vegetable oil
4 free-range eggs
1 avocado, cut into chunks
a few dashes of good Mexican
    chilli sauce (I love Cholula)

Heat the oil in a small frying pan. Add the garlic and chilli and fry for 1 minute, stirring, or until the garlic starts to soften and go golden. Add in the tomatoes, tomato purée, red-wine vinegar and half the coriander and cook over a medium-high heat for 9 minutes, until the tomatoes have reduced slightly. Season to taste and set aside.

Put the refried beans, if using, in a small saucepan and heat gently.

Meanwhile, heat a frying pan, add the tortillas and toast them for 20–30 seconds on each side. Remove from the pan and divide between plates. Pour the vegetable oil into the pan, add the eggs and fry for 1–2 minutes, basting the yolks with the hot oil as you go.

To serve, spread a spoonful of the refried beans between the tortillas, then dollop the tomato sauce on top. Top each plate of tortilla with a fried egg, scatter over the avocado chunks and coriander and finish with a little fiery chilli sauce.

SERVES: 2
PREPARATION TIME: 5 MINUTES
COOKING TIME: 10 MINUTES

WICKED RATING 5

BLACK Sticky RICE with Coconut & MANGO

Black glutinous rice is available in Asian supermarkets and makes the most wonderful rice-pudding-type porridge that can be eaten for breakfast or even for pudding after a south-east Asian meal. It's sticky, sweet, coconutty and, most of all, completely moreish. It takes a bit of time to cook the rice, so for a long, drawn-out Sunday morning brunch, whack it in a pot and leave it to cook for a couple of hours while you read the papers, or make it the night before if you want to wake up and eat it straight away.

100g black glutinous rice

400ml coconut water or ordinary water

sea salt

50g palm or muscovado sugar

1 x 400ml can coconut milk

1 fresh mango, cut into chunks

40g peanut brittle, roughly chopped

Put the rice, coconut water and a pinch of salt into a saucepan and bring to the boil, then reduce the heat to low and simmer, covered, for 45 minutes, until the rice is cooked through but is still wet.

Stir in the sugar, another pinch of salt, and 340ml of the coconut milk and bring to a boil. Reduce the heat to low and simmer, uncovered, stirring occasionally, until the mixture is thick and the rice is tender but still slightly chewy, about 30 minutes.

Remove the rice from the heat and leave for at least 30 minutes, stirring occasionally, until the rice has cooled to room temperature.

Just before serving, stir the rice and divide among 4 bowls. Drizzle over the remaining coconut milk and top with the mango and peanut brittle.

SERVES: 4
PREPARATION TIME: 10 MINUTES
COOKING TIME: 2 HOURS

WICKED RATING 5

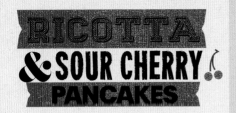

RICOTTA & SOUR CHERRY PANCAKES

250g ricotta cheese
2 free-range eggs, beaten
5 tbsp plain flour
½ tsp baking powder
2 tbsp sugar
1 tsp vanilla extract
200g fresh black sour
    cherries, pitted
1 tbsp olive oil
maple syrup, for serving

Ricotta pancakes, if you've never tried them, are so much lighter than regular pancakes, with an almost cheesecake-like texture. The ricotta and sour cherry combo comes from a gelato I had in Rome a few years back. The taste never really left me and, after making ricotta pancakes for the first time and trying to rack my brains as to what would work with them, I had this epiphany! Think along the lines of a grown-up blueberry pancake...

Put the ricotta in a large mixing bowl and beat until it is broken down and relatively smooth. Beat in the eggs one at a time, then add the flour, baking powder, sugar and vanilla and beat together to form a batter. (The batter will be a little lumpy because of the ricotta, but don't worry). Finally, gently stir in the cherries. They may bleed their juices into the batter a bit but this looks beautiful; just be careful not to over-stir.

Heat a pancake or frying pan over a medium heat. Dip a piece of kitchen paper into the oil and wipe around the pan. Drop a couple of tablespoons of batter into the pan to form a small pancake, then repeat to fit as many as you can comfortably in the pan (mine fits about 3–4).

Cook the pancakes for 1–2 minutes, or until the undersides are lightly browned. Flip them over and cook for another minute or so, until golden and cooked through. Slide the pancakes out of the pan and set aside on kitchen paper. Repeat until all the batter is used up. Serve hot with maple syrup.

SERVES: 2
PREPARATION TIME: 10 MINUTES
COOKING TIME: 10 MINUTES

WICKED RATING

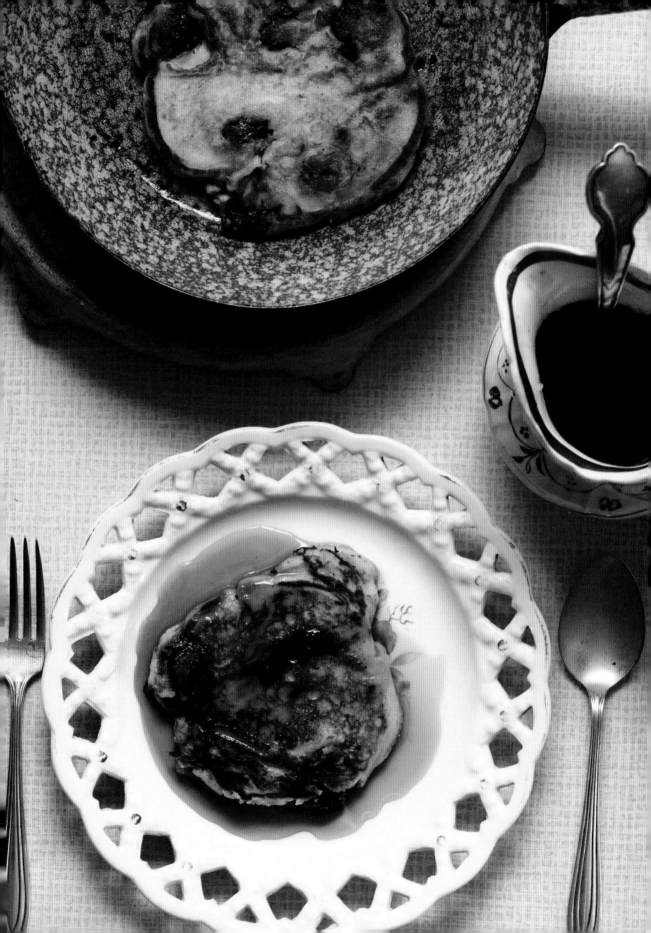

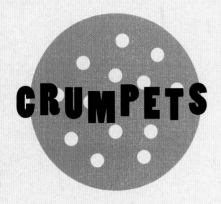

CRUMPETS

75ml boiling water
275ml whole milk
1 x 7g sachet fast-action dried
    yeast
1 tsp sugar
240g strong white bread flour
1 tsp baking powder
1 tsp fine salt
butter, for greasing and frying

GiZZi!! Tip

If you don't have crumpet
rings, just make these
like you would American
pancakes, spooning the
batter directly into the
pan. The only thing now
is that they are no longer
crumpets, and are called
pikelets instead!

MAKES: ABOUT
8 CRUMPETS
PREPARATION
TIME: 15 MINUTES
(PLUS A MINIMUM
1 HOUR PROVING TIME)
COOKING TIME:
15 MINUTES

WICKED RATING 8

Anyone who follows me on twitter will know I am
obsessed with making crumpets. It's a crumpet,
for God's sake: a crumpet! And you have made it
with your own fair hands. I don't really need to
explain any more that that, do I? This particular
recipe is the best I've tried and I totally stole it
from my really good pal, chef and food writer
Stevie Parle from the Dock Kitchen in London.
They are also served at his sister's café, The
Railroad in Hackney, which I frequent a little
too much. Like the best of us, the Parle family
clearly loves a bit of crumpet...

Pour the boiling water and milk into a bowl, stir in the
yeast and sugar and leave to sit somewhere warm for
15 minutes.

Sieve the flour into a mixing bowl with the baking
powder and salt. Slowly add the milk and yeast mix,
whisking as you do so to create a thick batter. Cover
with clingfilm and leave to prove for at least an hour.
(I often make this before bed and leave it covered in
the fridge overnight – by morning it's perfect.)

Gently heat a large, heavy frying pan and add a
knob of butter. Grease 2 crumpet rings well. Set them
in the pan, then, with a big spoon, carefully scoop the
mixture into each until three-quarters full.

Cook the crumpets over a low heat for about 5–8
minutes, or until the crumpet batter is set all the
way to the top. Remove the crumpet rings, flip the
crumpets over and finish the tops so that they are
nicely browned. Whack them straight onto a plate
and slather them in lots of salted butter. Serve with
tea and the papers.

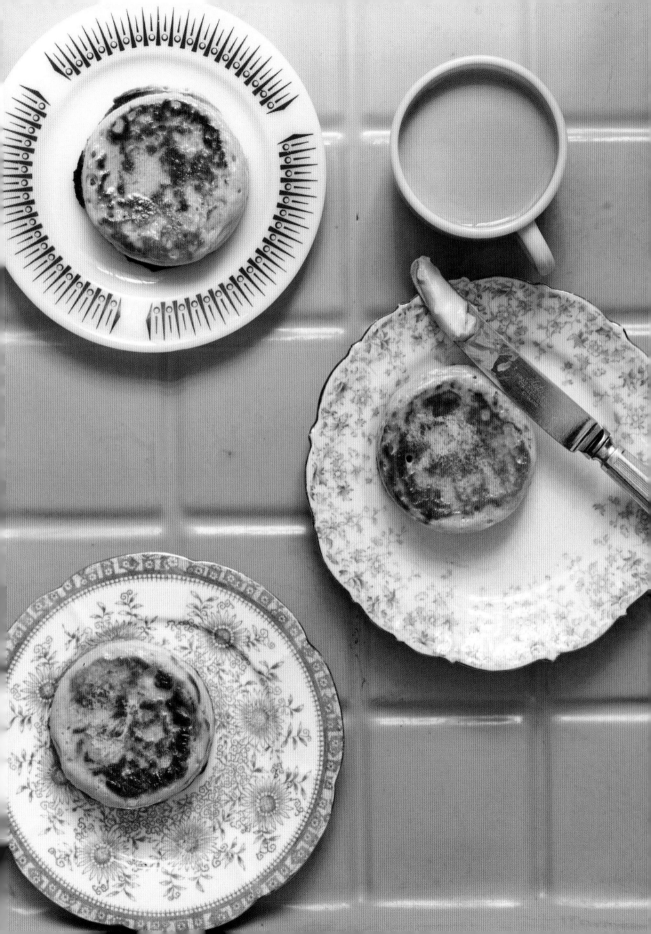

SUNDAY LUNCH

AKA
THE BIG
SHEBANG

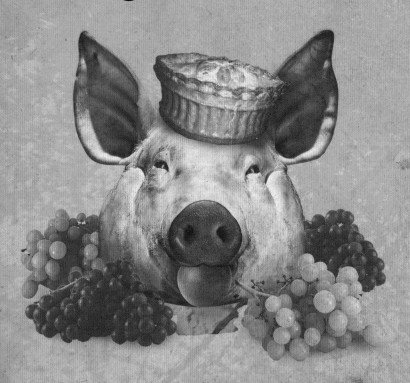

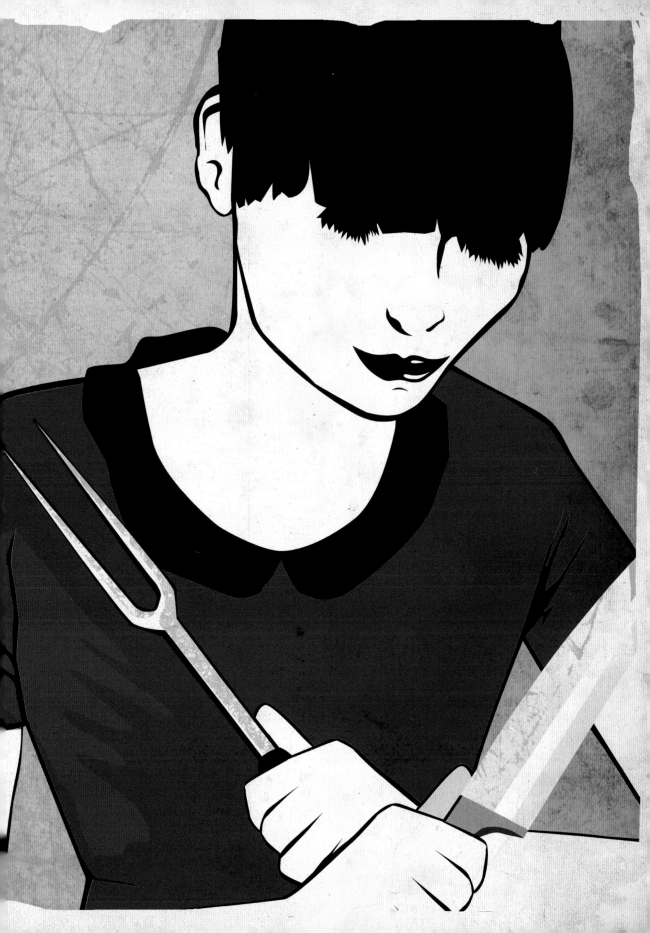

Tomato water WITH THAI BASIL, TOMATO PETALS AND RATATOUILLE

• • • • • • • • •

I first made this soup for Boy George and Adam Ant at a supper club I did and everyone went wild for it. Making the tomato water itself is a slow process but the results are beautiful and it's packed full of flavour. Lightly sautéed vegetables and tomato petals are added to this fragrant tomato water, with the whole lot finished off with Thai basil to give it a little aniseed kick at the end. So, so delicious.

6 vine-ripened tomatoes
a handful of Thai basil or basil
    cress leaves, to serve

For the tomato water
3kg mixed plum and
    cherry tomatoes
2 garlic cloves
16 basil leaves
2 tsp sea salt
1 tsp sugar

For the ratatouille
1 tbsp olive oil, plus extra
    for drizzling
1 large aubergine, finely chopped
1 green courgette,
    finely chopped
1 yellow courgette or small
    summer squash, finely chopped
1 vine-ripened tomato, peeled,
    deseeded and finely chopped
sea salt and freshly ground
    black pepper

To make the tomato water, put all the ingredients in a liquidiser and blend to a chunky purée. Pour into a muslin-lined sieve set over a large bowl. Transfer to the fridge and leave for 3–4 hours to drip slowly through the muslin and chill.

For the tomato petals, make a cross in the bottom of each tomato with a knife and pop in a bowl. Cover with boiling water and leave to sit for a minute. Remove with a slotted spoon and cool, then peel the skin off with your fingers. Cut each tomato into eighths and scrape out the seeds with a teaspoon. Set aside.

To make the ratatouille, heat the oil in a pan, add the aubergine and fry for 1–2 minutes. Add the courgettes and cook for a further 2–3 minutes, until the veg are cooked through but not coloured. Add the tomato and cook for another minute, until the pieces start to break down. Season and set aside.

To serve, arrange the tomato petals artfully in soup bowls and place the ratatouille in the centre of each. Carefully ladle in the tomato water, drizzle with olive oil and scatter over the basil leaves to finish.

SERVES: 6
PREPARATION TIME: 4 HOURS
COOKING TIME: 10 MINUTES

WICKED RATING 1

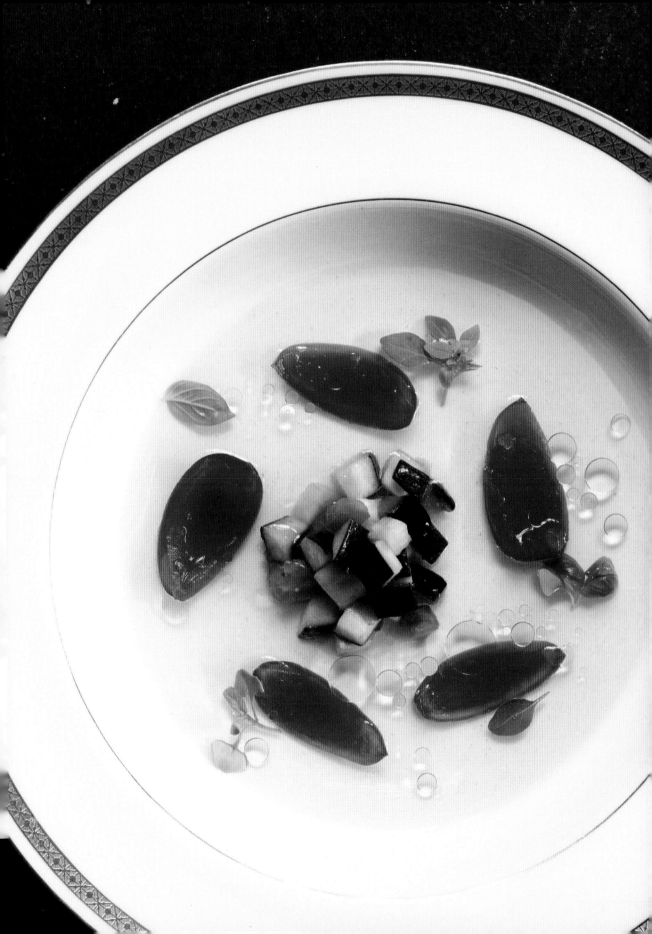

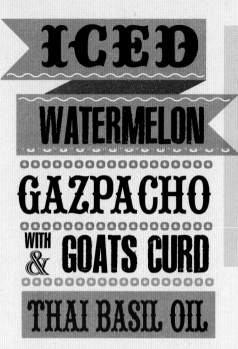

ICED WATERMELON GAZPACHO WITH & GOATS CURD THAI BASIL OIL

There is a running joke in my family about my mother and her fruit soups. When I was a kid she used to serve them as a starter at her dinner parties and me and my sisters used to roll around the floor in hysterics thinking she was totally barking! Oh, how the tables have turned. I now love serving fruit soups. This watermelon gazpacho goes so well with the fresh goat's curd and Thai basil oil as a really light starter that's so easy to whip up after a hard day's work.

1kg watermelon, peeled
    and deseeded
½ red pepper, chopped
½ cucumber, peeled and
    chopped
2 shallots, chopped
a small handful of fresh
    basil
½ tsp sea salt
2 tbsp extra-virgin olive oil,
    plus extra for drizzling
3 tbsp red-wine vinegar
a handful or two of ice cubes
4 tbsp fresh goat's curd
a small handful of micro basil or
    Thai basil leaves, to serve

For the Thai basil oil
a handful of basil leaves
a handful of Thai basil leaves
    (or another of ordinary basil)
4 tbsp extra-virgin olive oil
the juice of ½ a lemon
sea salt and freshly ground
    black pepper

Take 100g of the watermelon, finely dice it and set aside. Pop the remaining watermelon, red pepper, cucumber, shallots, basil, salt, olive oil and vinegar into a blender and blitz until smooth. Lay two bits of plain kitchen paper over a sieve, add the liquid and strain, reserving the liquid that comes though the sieve and discarding what remains in it. Pour the reserved liquid into a jug with the ice cubes and set aside in the fridge.

To make the oil, put both basils, the oil, lemon juice and a little salt and pepper into the blender and blitz until smooth. Strain through a sieve and set aside.

Carefully shape the goat's curd between two hot spoons into quenelles and divide among 6 shallow soup bowls.

Scatter the diced watermelon into the bowls around the quenelles, then carefully pour the watermelon gazpacho into the bowls so as not to break up the curd. Drizzle each bowl with half a teaspoon of the basil oil and scatter over a few basil leaves to finish.

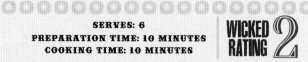

SERVES: 6
PREPARATION TIME: 10 MINUTES
COOKING TIME: 10 MINUTES

WICKED RATING 2

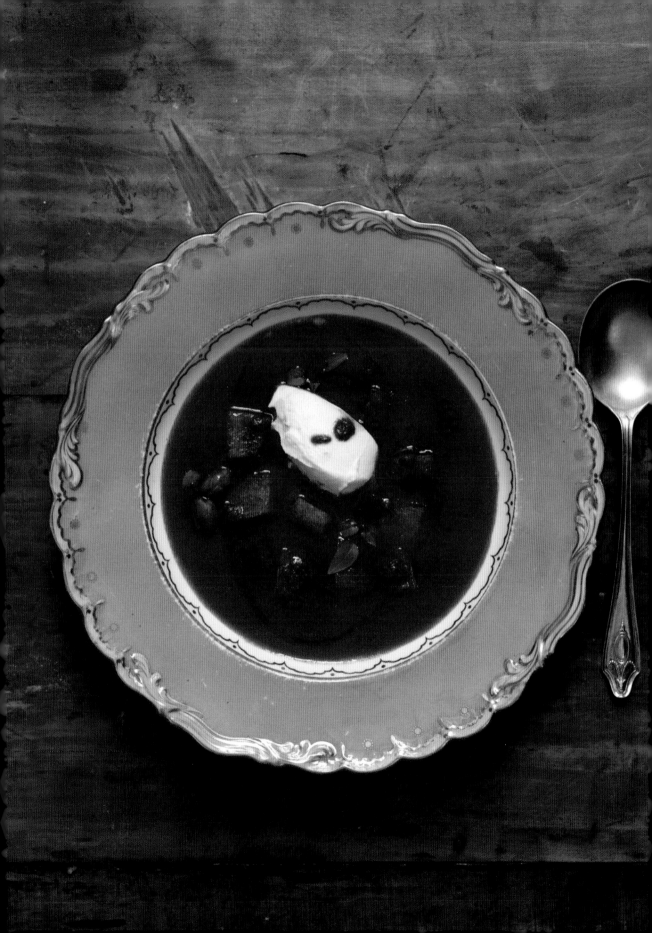

BEEF CARPACCIO WITH GORGONZOLA, CANDIED NUTS & ROCKET

I'm not normally one to fix something that ain't broke, and carpaccio is one of those things whose purity is its selling point: a simple drizzle of oil, a squeeze of lemon and a pinch of salt turn raw beef into a thing of beauty. But this recipe was born in unusual circumstances, and I'm so glad it was – the result of having some delicious Gorgonzola dolce in my fridge that I had got in to make something else. I thought I'd just see how it went with the raw meat and...well, my God, it was good.

500g beef fillet (you'll need a nice thick piece of centre cut)
sea salt and freshly ground black pepper
juice of ½ a lemon
good-quality olive oil, for drizzling
160g Gorgonzola dolce, cubed
50g rocket leaves

For the candied nuts
60g caster sugar
100g walnuts

For the dressing
100g Gorgonzola dolce, cubed
100ml sour cream
juice of 1 lemon

First things first: put the beef into the freezer for 1–2 hours to firm it up and make it easier to slice. (It should not be frozen as such, just really firm).

Next, get on with the nuts. Melt the sugar in a dry frying pan until it starts to caramelise. Quickly pop the nuts into the pan and coat them in the caramel. Turn them out onto greaseproof paper and leave to dry.

To make the dressing, pop the ingredients into a blender and blitz until smooth. Season and set aside.

Take the beef out of the freezer. Using a very sharp, large knife, slice the beef as finely as possible. Divide the slices among 6 plates and arrange them as you like. Scatter over a little sea salt and black pepper, squeeze over the lemon juice and drizzle with some really good olive oil.

If you have a chef's bottle, load your dressing with it and use it to do some cheffy zigzags all over the meat. (If you don't have one, just drizzle or smear the dressing over the meat any which way you like.)

Roughly chop the walnuts and dot them and the cheese among the plates. Dress the salad leaves with a little more olive oil and lemon juice and arrange on top of the carpaccio.

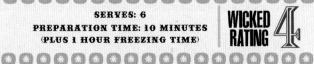

SERVES: 6
PREPARATION TIME: 10 MINUTES
(PLUS 1 HOUR FREEZING TIME)

WICKED RATING 4

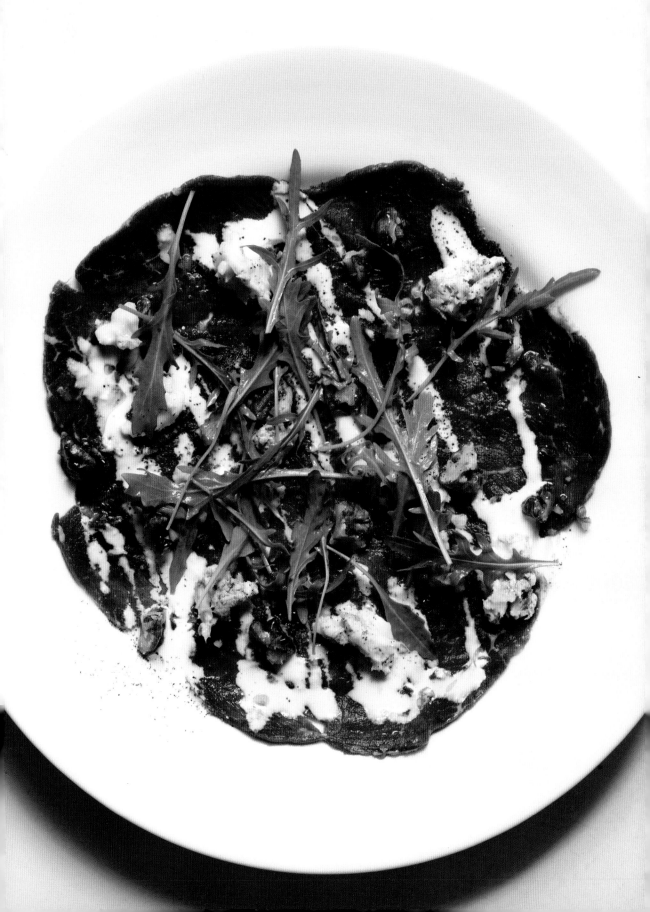

SALMON TARTARE WITH CHILLI, CAPERS, ROCKET, & LEMON

This is nothing like steak tartare, I just can't think of a better way to describe it! I've taken raw salmon and paired it with some classically Italian ingredients to make an easy, fresh and light way to start a meal. If you're a bit funny about raw fish or cooking with raw fish at home, this is just as delicious with those thick smoked salmon Tsar fillets.

900g really fresh salmon fillet, skin removed
3 red chillies, finely chopped
3 tbsp capers (in vinegar), chopped
2 tsp sea salt
juice of 4 lemons
3 tbsp olive oil
50g rocket leaves

Place the salmon fillet on a clean chopping board and chop into 7mm cubes with a sharp knife (it's important to try and keep these pieces the same size).

Pop the salmon pieces in a large mixing bowl with the remaining ingredients. Give everything a really good mix together and then divide between plates or arrange on a serving platter. Eat immediately.

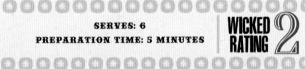

SERVES: 6
PREPARATION TIME: 5 MINUTES

WICKED RATING 2

HOT ARTICHOKE DIP

1 x 170g jar of grilled artichoke hearts
40g Parmesan, grated
1 garlic clove, grated
250ml double cream
1 free-range egg yolk
a good pinch of cayenne pepper
a squeeze of lemon juice
sea salt and freshly ground black pepper

The first time I had this was at an American steakhouse on Park Lane. It blew my mind. Since then I've had the real deal in steakhouses all over New York and boy, is it moreish. Served alongside a whole load of crudités and good breads, it makes a wonderfully wicked counterpart to the skinny dips that feature earlier in this book.

Heat the oven to 200ºC/Gas 6.

Drain the artichokes well. (I'd even go so far as to say to pat them dry with kitchen paper, as they can be a little wet from the jar.) Pop them in a blender with the rest of the ingredients and blend for about 1 minute, until really smooth.

Transfer the mix to an ovenproof dish and bake for 20–25 minutes, or until piping hot and nicely golden on top. Remove from the oven and serve straight away with bread and crudités for dipping.

SERVES 6
PREPARATION TIME: 10 MINUTES
COOKING TIME: 20–25 MINUTES

 WICKED RATING 4

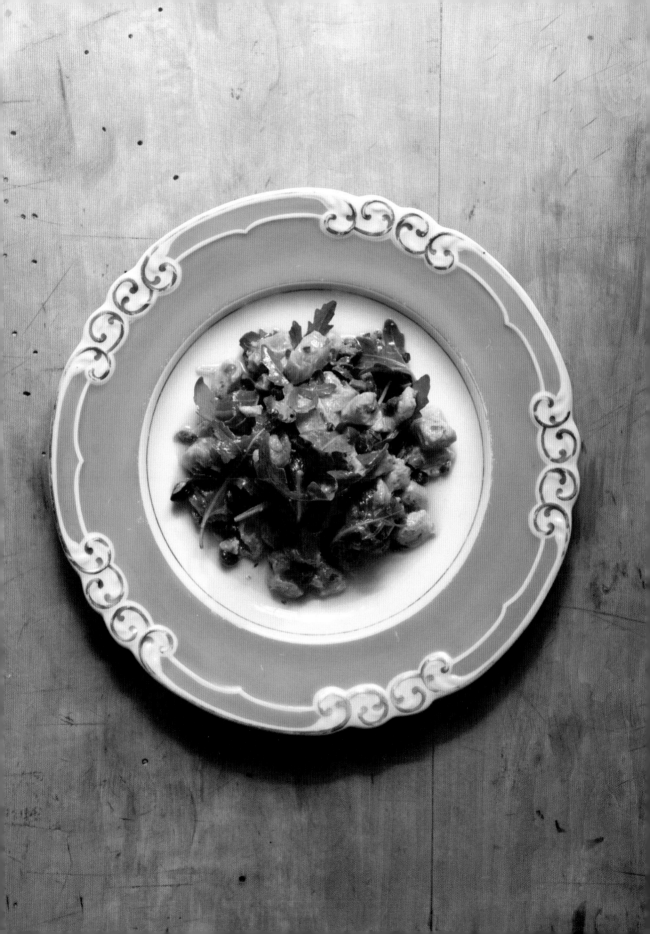

PINK DEVILLED eggs with BAKED BABY BEET SALAD

Pickled eggs are back! And with the continuing resurgence of traditional British food, we'll be seeing a lot more of them. But these eggs are not at all like the ones we grew up with. Instead, they are softer boiled and only pickled for a matter of days in a beetroot liquor that gives them both a great flavour and a beautiful colour. Served with roasted multicoloured beets, they make quite the swanky starter.

For the eggs

9 free-range eggs (try and invest in Cotswold legbars or Burford browns, as their really yellow yolks will look extra-beautiful)
4 raw beetroot
150ml water, plus extra for blitzing
80g golden caster sugar
sea salt
a couple of peppercorns
1 onion, thinly sliced
4 tbsp mayonnaise
a good pinch of cayenne pepper
a good pinch of paprika

For the salad

500g mixed coloured beetroot (the smaller the better)
50g frisée lettuce
40g base dressing (see page 36)

Lower the eggs gently into a pan of boiling water and leave to boil for 8–9 minutes. Remove and run under cold water, then peel carefully. Set aside in a bowl.

If you have a juicer, juice the beetroot. If you don't, blitz them in a food processor with a couple of tablespoons of water, then sieve out the juice, discarding the pithy bits. Set aside.

Heat the water, sugar, 1 tablespoon of salt, peppercorns and onion in a saucepan, stirring, until the sugar melts. Add the beetroot juice and stir to combine. Pour the liquid over the boiled eggs, cover with clingfilm and leave in the fridge for between 12 to 24 hours. Give them a stir halfway through the pickling process – the eggs will be bright pink when they are ready.

To make the salad, preheat the oven to 190ºC/ Gas 5. Individually wrap the beetroot in foil, adding a sprinkling of salt to each. Bake for 40 minutes, or until just tender. Remove from the oven and leave to cool. Cut larger beetroot into 1cm cubes (tiny ones can be halved or quartered instead).

Halve the eggs, scoop out the yolks and pop into a bowl. Lay the empty egg whites on a tray. Add the mayo, cayenne, paprika and a pinch of salt to the bowl and mash them until they become a smooth paste. Refill the egg whites with the yolk paste using a piping bag or spoon.

Mix the dressing together with the lettuce and beets, then split between plates. Top with 3 egg halves per plate and serve.

SERVES: 6
PREPARATION TIME: 10 MINUTES (PLUS A MINIMUM 12 HOURS PICKLING TIME)
COOKING TIME: 40 MINUTES

WICKED RATING 3

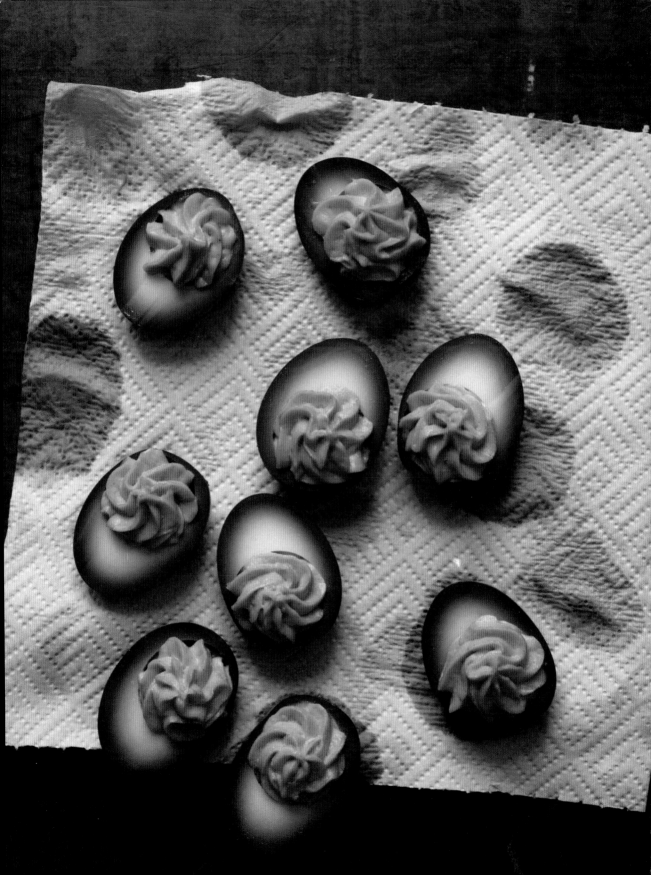

ROAST CHICKEN with TRUFFLED GNOCCHI & sage butter

Don't get me wrong: I love a classic chicken with all the sides, but sometimes it's nice to get something a bit more from your roast. Gnocchi are so fun to make and crazy good smothered in this truffle-spiked brown butter with sage. A sophisticated change to the old classic.

1 tbsp butter mixed with 3 chopped sage leaves
1 x 2kg organic chicken
sea salt and freshly ground black pepper
100g cavolo nero, or other seasonal cabbage, shredded

For the truffled gnocchi
250g evenly sized floury potatoes, baked and still hot
50g Italian '00' flour, plus extra for dusting
¼ tsp fine sea salt
25g Parmesan, finely grated, plus extra for serving
1 tsp white truffle paste or white truffle oil
1 egg yolk, lightly beaten

For the sage and truffle butter
30g unsalted butter
a handful of sage leaves
1–2 tsp truffle-infused olive oil

Preheat the oven to 220°C/Gas 7. Rub the sage butter under the chicken skin, season with salt and roast for 20 minutes. Lower the oven to 190°C/Gas 5 and cook for 1 hour, or until the juices run clear. Cover with foil and leave to rest.

Meanwhile, make the gnocchi. Scoop the flesh out of the baked potatoes and mash using a potato ricer into a large mixing bowl. Form a well in the centre of the mashed potato, add the flour, salt and cheese and stir together, then gradually mix in the truffle paste and beaten egg. Press the mixture together to form a dough, adding a little more flour if it seems too wet, and tip onto a floured surface. Shape into a long log, then cut into 2cm lengths. Using a fork, press down onto the top of each, then gently squeeze the sides so that the gnocchi resemble pillows.

For the sage and truffle butter, put the butter and sage in a small pan and cook over a medium heat until the butter is golden brown and smelling nutty. Remove from the heat and stir in the truffle oil.

Bring a pan of salted water to the boil, add the gnocchi and cavolo nero and cook for 1–2 minutes, or until the gnocchi have risen to the surface. Strain, add to the butter sauce and fry until the gnocchi are coated and catching in places. Carve or portion the chicken and arrange the gnocchi and cavolo nero on plates. Pile the chicken on top and spoon over the chicken juices from the tin to finish.

SERVES: 6
PREPARATION TIME: 30 MINUTES
COOKING TIME: 90 MINUTES

 WICKED RATING 7

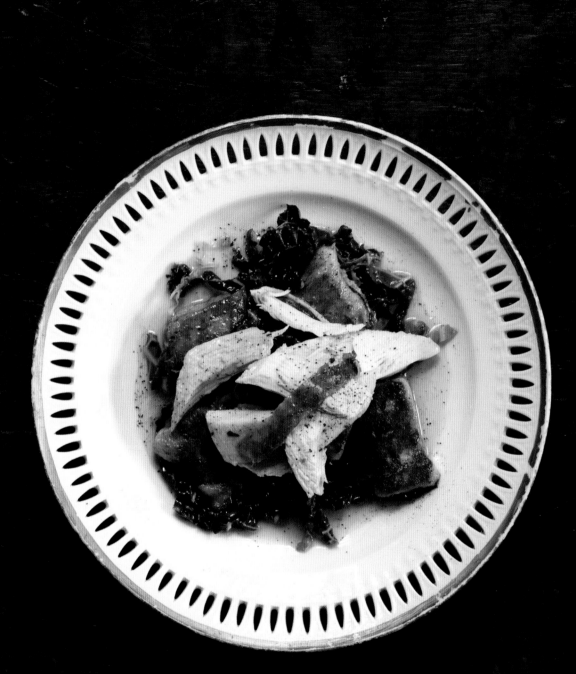

SLOW-ROASTED POMEGRANATE DUCK WITH POTATO CAKES & CHICORY

I'm not claiming dibs on the whole duck-and-pomegranate thing. I first read about it in the Moro cookbook and spent ages playing with the combination – using griddled quail, guinea fowl and lamb – but the sharpness of the pomegranate slices brilliantly through the fattiness of the duck and it really is the best. Here I've given the combination a bit of an Anglo twist, slow-roasting the duck to turn it into an exceptional Sunday lunch.

1 x 2kg duck (look out for a big-busted number), excess skin trimmed and giblets removed
1 tsp Chinese five-spice powder
sea salt and freshly ground black pepper
1 tbsp plain flour
400ml chicken stock
a sprig of thyme
2 tbsp pomegranate molasses
a pinch of cinnamon
a pinch of allspice

For the potato cake
50g melted duck fat (I drain this off the duck after 30 minutes cooking)
1 tsp thyme leaves
800g floury potatoes, peeled and very finely sliced with a mandolin or sharp knife

For the chicory
1 tsp olive oil
1 tsp butter
3–4 heads of chicory, cut in half lengthways
150ml chicken stock mixed with 1 tbsp pomegranate molasses
a few sprigs of thyme

Heat the oven to 200°C/Gas 6. Score the skin on the duck breast in a crosshatch pattern, then prick all over. Rub with the five-spice and a little salt and pepper, then place breast-side up on the wire rack of a large roasting pan and cook for 20 minutes. Lower the heat to 170°C/Gas 3, turn over carefully and cook for 45 minutes, then turn breast-side up again and cook for a final 45 minutes. Cover with foil and leave to rest for 15 minutes before carving.

Meanwhile, make the potato cake. Grease a 20cm sandwich tin with the fat, then sprinkle with salt and thyme. Lay a layer of potato slices neatly overlapping each other on the base of the tin in concentric circles.

Layer the rest of the potatoes in the same way, seasoning with salt and pepper every 2 layers. Cook in the oven for 1 hour 15 minutes, until crisp on the outside and soft in the centre. Turn onto a board and sprinkle with a little more salt.

For the chicory, heat the oil and butter in a pan until foaming, add the chicory and fry for 3–4 minutes, turning halfway, until golden brown. Lay the pieces cut-side up in a baking dish and pour over the stock. Season and sprinkle over the thyme. Bake for 30 minutes.

Warm the roasting juices over a medium heat, pouring off any excess fat. Whisk in the flour and cook for 1 minute, then slowly add the stock, whisking, until combined. Add the thyme and cook until reduced, then add the molasses and spices and season to taste. Carve the duck and serve with the gravy, potato cake and baked chicory.

SERVES: 6
PREPARATION TIME: 15 MINUTES
COOKING TIME: 3 HOURS

WICKED RATING 8

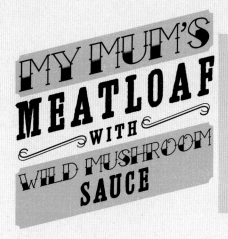

MY MUM'S MEATLOAF WITH WILD MUSHROOM SAUCE

My mum was always a creative cook, but in some cases that came out of necessity. Often she would make us a regular meatloaf for Sunday lunches, but when entertaining she would 'zhoosh it up' with wild mushrooms and tarragon. It's a delicious dish, and one that I'm actually very proud is finally getting out there.

1 tsp butter, plus extra
    for greasing
1 large onion, finely chopped
2 garlic cloves, finely chopped
a few sprigs of fresh thyme, leaves
    pulled off and chopped
2 sprigs of rosemary, leaves
    pulled and finely chopped
400g beef mince
200g pork mince
100g fresh white breadcrumbs
2 egg yolks
a splash of milk
a pinch of nutmeg
sea salt and freshly ground
    black pepper

For the sauce
1 tsp butter
1 tsp rapeseed or olive oil
300g seasonal wild or chestnut
    mushrooms
150g small fresh porcini or
    morels, sliced (or the same
    volume of rehydrated porcini)
2 garlic cloves, finely chopped
1 tsp plain flour
400ml beef stock
a splash of Madeira or Marsala
100ml double cream
a few sprigs of tarragon,
    leaves only
zest of ½ a lemon

Preheat the oven to 220°C/Gas 7. Melt the butter in a small frying pan until foaming. Add the onion and sauté gently for around 10 minutes, until softened and lightly golden. Stir in the garlic, thyme and rosemary and cook for a further minute. Remove from the heat and set aside for 5–10 minutes to cool.

In a bowl, mix together the beef and pork mince, breadcrumbs, egg yolks, milk, cooked onions and nutmeg and season well. Shape the mixture into a loaf shape and place on a greased roasting tray. Put in the oven and roast for 20 minutes, then lower the temperature to 180°C/Gas 4 and cook for a further 30 minutes, until golden brown. Remove from the oven, cover with foil and leave to rest for 10 minutes.

To make the sauce, put the roasting tray over a medium-high heat and add the butter. Once the butter is foaming, add the mushrooms and fry for 2–3 minutes, or until golden, scraping up all the sticky bits from the bottom of the tray as you go. Add the garlic and sweat for 1 minute, then add the flour and mix to form a thick paste. Pour in the stock and booze, stirring, and leave to bubble away until reduced by about two-thirds. Pour in the cream, then add the tarragon, lemon zest and season with salt and pepper. Continue to cook until the sauce has reduced to a creamy pouring consistency.

Slice up the meatloaf and arrange on plates. Pour over the mushroom sauce and serve with creamy mash.

SERVES: 6
PREPARATION
TIME: 15 MINUTES
COOKING TIME:
1 HOUR

WICKED RATING 7

Korean ROAST LAMB SHOULDER

Korean barbecue is hot right now, but quite hard to recreate at home. By marinating a lamb shoulder in the same Korean flavours of soy, miso, gochujang (Korean chilli paste) and sesame and then letting it cook till it falls off the bone you'll have the perfect meat to wrap up in lettuce with sticky sushi rice, cucumber, spring onions, hoisin and sriracha (the very trendy Asian hot sauce). It's a great alternative to the classic Sunday lunch, but still gives you the satisfaction of having a big hunk of meat roasting away for hours!

6 garlic cloves, grated
4 spring onions, finely chopped
a thumb-sized piece of ginger, grated
3 tbsp sesame oil
2 tbsp gochujang
4 tbsp sweet white miso paste
2 tbsp soy sauce
1 tbsp mirin
1 x 1.5kg lamb shoulder
sea salt and freshly ground black pepper
2 tbsp vegetable oil

To serve
a head of romaine lettuce
4 spring onions, finely julienned
1 cucumber, deseeded and finely julienned
360g sushi rice, cooked according to the packet instructions
2–3 tbsp toasted sesame seeds
hoisin sauce
sriracha (Asian chilli sauce)

Mix together the garlic, spring onions, ginger, sesame oil, gochujang, miso, soy and mirin. Season the lamb shoulder with salt and pepper, then smother with the marinade. Cover with clingfilm and leave to marinate for 2 hours.

Heat the oven to 200°C/Gas 6. Heat the vegetable oil in a roasting tin. Remove the meat from the marinade, add to the tin and brown on all sides. (The meat will catch slightly because of the sugar in the marinade, so be mindful of this.) Transfer the browned lamb to the oven and roast for 30 minutes. Lower the temperature to 170°C/Gas 3 and roast for another 3 hours, or until the lamb is falling off the bone.

Carefully transfer the lamb onto a serving plate. Tip the excess fat from the pan and spoon the remaining juices over the meat. Use a couple of forks to pull the lamb meat into shreds. Arrange the lettuce leaves, spring onions, and cucumber on separate plates. Pop the rice in a serving bowl and top with the sesame seeds.

To eat, fill a lettuce leaf with a small spoonful of rice, a few spring onions and a dollop each of hoisin sauce and sriracha. Top with the shredded lamb, wrap and munch.

SERVES: 8
PREPARATION TIME: 10 MINUTES (PLUS 2 HOURS MARINATING TIME)
COOKING TIME: 4 HOURS

WICKED RATING 6

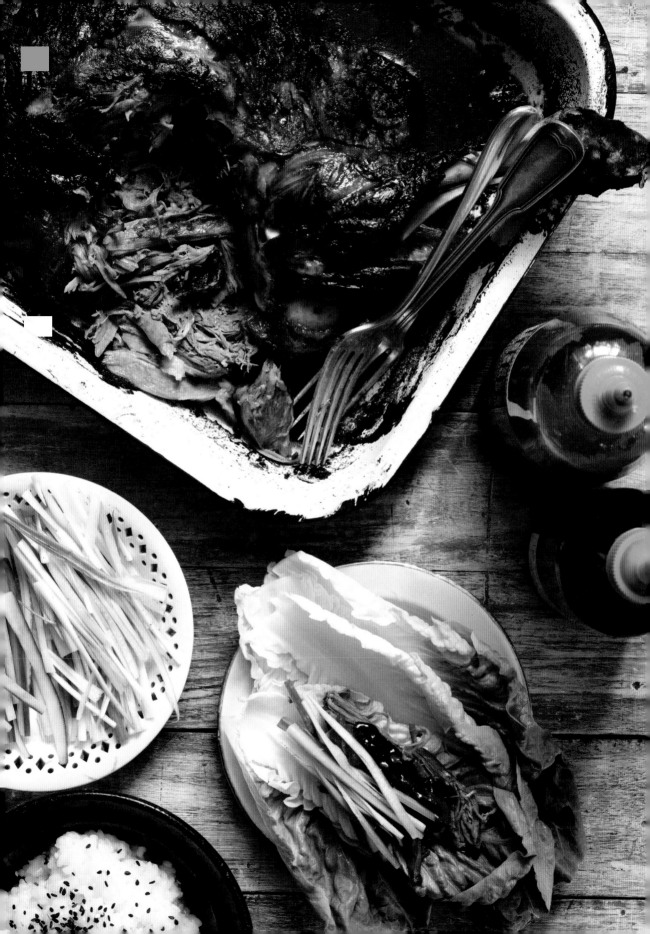

BRAISED VEAL SHIN
BOURGUIGNON

2–3kg rose veal shin
sea salt and freshly ground
    black pepper
2 tbsp olive oil
150g smoked streaky bacon
15 shallots, peeled
8 garlic cloves, peeled but left
    whole
1 tsp tomato purée
1 tbsp plain flour
a bottle of good red wine
200ml Port (optional)
500ml fresh veal or beef stock
1 bay leaf
a few sprigs of thyme
2 cloves
4 carrots, peeled and cut in half
    lengthways
400g chestnut mushrooms,
    halved

Boeuf bourguignon is up there as one of my dream comfort suppers, but there's no reason we can't make it into a more Sunday roast kind of a deal. Braising the whole shin of veal very slowly until it falls off the bone into the braising liquor of smoky bacon, mushrooms, shallots, carrots and red wine makes for a delicious Sunday lunch and, if you're a bone-marrow fan like me, you get to spread the bone marrow on grilled bread as a starter! You could use beef shin for this but we need to be eating more veal. Veal has had such a stigma attached to it largely because of the Dutch milk-fed kind, but the stuff labelled rose veal is treated very well and I think it's better to eat it than not – useless for meat in adulthood, male dairy cows are often disposed of unless they're eaten, which is a terrible waste. So go on: give veal a go.

Heat the oven to 170ºC/Gas 3. Rub the veal shin with salt and pepper. Heat the oil in a large casserole into which the veal shin will fit easily. Add the veal and brown on all sides, about 7 minutes. Remove from the pan and set aside.

Lower the heat, add the bacon to the casserole and cook, scraping up all the sticky bits from the bottom of the tray as you go, until the bacon is turning golden and crisp. Add the shallots and garlic and cook, stirring, for a minute or two. Add the tomato purée and cook, stirring, for 30 seconds, then add the flour and cook off for a further 30 seconds. Gradually pour in the wine, then the Port and veal or beef stock.

Pop the shin back into the pan with the herbs and cloves, put the lid on and put into the oven. Roast for 5 hours. Remove from the oven, add the carrots and cook for a further 30 minutes. Add the mushrooms. The meat is ready when it is falling from the bone and the sauce is rich and a little reduced.

Remove the casserole from the oven and leave to rest for 15 minutes before serving (this resting time will make pulling the meat from the bone a little easier). Serve with toasted bread spread with paté, good mash, or roasties, Yorkshire puds and all the trimmings if you'd prefer.

SERVES: 6
PREPARATION
TIME: 30 MINUTES
COOKING TIME:
6 HOURS

WICKED RATING 8

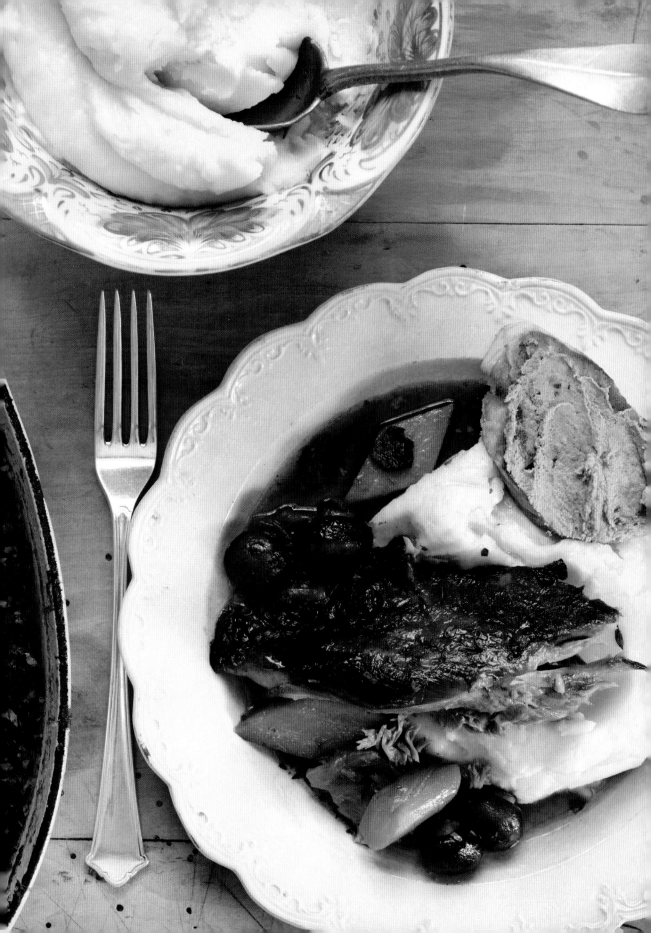

VENISON WELLINGTON

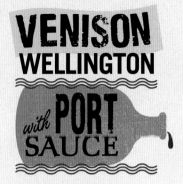

with PORT SAUCE

We should all be eating more venison. I can't begin to tell you how delicious it is, but it's also so good for you as it's really lean, super-ethical as it's not farmed and to top it off, it's good value. My favourite way to eat it is in this Wellington, paired with a sweet Port sauce. Served with greens and a proper mash, it's a real Sunday lunch showstopper.

2 tbsp olive oil
sea salt and freshly ground
    black pepper
1 x 1kg well-trimmed boned
    venison loin fillet
2 banana shallots, finely
    chopped
5 portobello mushrooms, very
    finely chopped
5 chestnut mushrooms, very
    finely chopped
3 garlic cloves, finely chopped
a few fresh thyme sprigs
1 tsp truffle oil (optional)
12 slices of Parma ham
flour, for dusting
1 x 320g packet of ready-rolled,
    all-butter puff pastry
2 large free-range egg yolks,
    beaten

For the port sauce:
a knob of butter
1 large banana shallot, sliced
a sprig of thyme
300ml Port
500ml fresh beef stock
a few juniper berries

Heat 1 tablespoon of oil in a frying pan. Season the venison well, add to the pan and brown all over, about 5 minutes. Set aside to cool. Add the remaining oil and shallots to the pan and cook for 2 minutes, then add the mushrooms and fry for a further 10 minutes, or until they have softened and browned. Add the garlic, thyme and truffle oil and cook for 1 minute, then remove from the heat and leave to cool.

Lay out a double layer of clingfilm about 40cm long, then lay another double layer above it, overlapping the first by about 10cm so that you have a large rectangular grid of film. Starting at the bottom, lay 6 slices of Parma ham centrally, overlapping each slice with the next. Lay the next 6 slices in the same way above this layer to double the width. Spread the mushrooms over the ham. Place the venison at one end of the ham then, with the help of the clingfilm, roll the venison in the ham. Wrap the clingfilm round the venison and roll it tight, tying the ends like a cracker. Pop into the fridge for 30 minutes.

Roll the pastry out on a floured board into a 40cm x 30cm rectangle. Carefully unravel the ham-wrapped venison from the clingfilm and lay it along one of the long sides of the pastry. Roll the venison in the pastry. Trim off any excess from the sides and tuck the pastry under the meat.

Cut any excess pastry into shapes (I'm a fan of stars). Using a pastry brush, brush the beaten egg yolk over the pastry. Place the pastry shapes on top of the pastry, and then glaze these. Pop the Wellington into the fridge for 30 minutes. Preheat the oven to 200°C/Gas 6.

SERVES: 6
PREPARATION TIME:
1 HOUR 30 MINUTES
COOKING TIME:
45 MINUTES

WICKED RATING 8

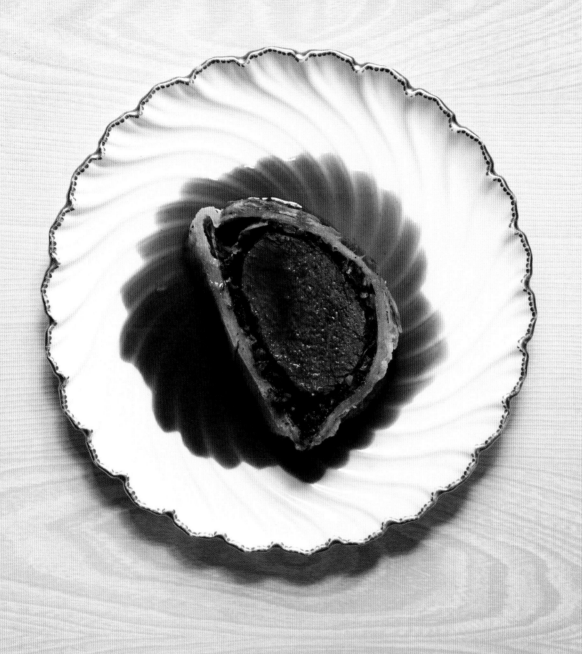

Remove from the fridge and bake for 25–30 minutes, or until the pastry has become golden and crisp, which indicates that the venison is cooked through perfectly and will be medium-rare. Leave to rest for 15 minutes.

Meanwhile, make the Port sauce. Put the butter in a pan, add the shallot and thyme and sweat gently. Pour in the port, bring to the boil and reduce by two-thirds, then add the beef stock and juniper berries and reduce again by two-thirds until syrupy. Strain and serve with the Wellington.

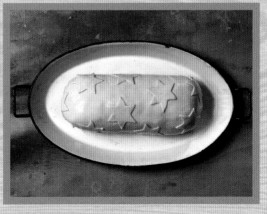

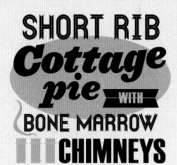

SHORT RIB
Cottage pie WITH
BONE MARROW
‖‖‖ CHIMNEYS

I first had this when I went to my friend Adam Byatt's restaurant Trinity, in Clapham, London and fell head over heels in love with it. With its braised short ribs and super-rich gelatinous stew, it was an instant win as far as I was concerned, so I pinched the recipe and I've made it my own. It's a meat-eater's heaven and a real showpiece for the table.

2 tbsp olive oil
2kg short ribs
sea salt and freshly ground
    black pepper
4 onions, finely chopped
2 carrots, peeled and roughly
    chopped
1 leek, roughly chopped
1 garlic bulb
1 star anise
1 tsp tomato purée
1 tbsp plain flour
400ml red wine
100ml Port
1 ½ litres fresh beef stock
a few sprigs of thyme,
    leaves only
3 sprigs of rosemary, leaves finely
    chopped, plus 3 extra
    sprigs to garnish
1 bay leaf
3 x 10cm beef marrowbones

For the mashed
    potato topping
1 ½ kg large floury potatoes,
    peeled, cut into pieces
    and boiled in salted water
    until tender
100ml milk
125g unsalted butter
sea salt and freshly ground
    black pepper

SERVES: 6
PREPARATION TIME:
30 MINUTES
COOKING TIME:
4 HOURS

WICKED RATING 9

Heat 1 tablespoon of olive oil in a large casserole dish. Season the ribs with salt and pepper, add to the pan and fry until browned on all sides. Remove from the pan and place on a wire rack suspended over a plate.

Add the onions, carrots, leek, garlic and star anise to the casserole and fry for 4–5 minutes, or until golden brown. Add the tomato purée and cook for another minute, then add the flour and stir to coat the veg. Add the red wine and Port, bring to the boil, then reduce to a simmer.

Return the ribs to the pan, add the stock and herbs and bring back to the boil, then simmer gently for three hours, or until the meat is falling off the bone. Remove the meat from the casserole and leave to cool.

Bring the remaining liquid to the boil and reduce until syrupy and rich-tasting. Meanwhile, shred the meat from the bones, discarding any fat and sinew. Return the shredded meat to the pan and take off the heat.

For the mash, pass the cooked potatoes through a ricer into a bowl. Bring the milk and butter to a simmer in a pan, then add to the potatoes and beat together well. Season and tip into a piping bag, snipping the end 3cm up.

Preheat the oven to 200°C/Gas 6. Spoon the meat stew into a large ovenproof dish and arrange the marrowbone pieces around the centre, placing a rosemary sprig in the top of each. Pipe the mash onto the meat in little turrets and cook in the oven for 30–40 minutes, or until golden and bubbling. Serve with peas and a little Worcestershire sauce, if you like.

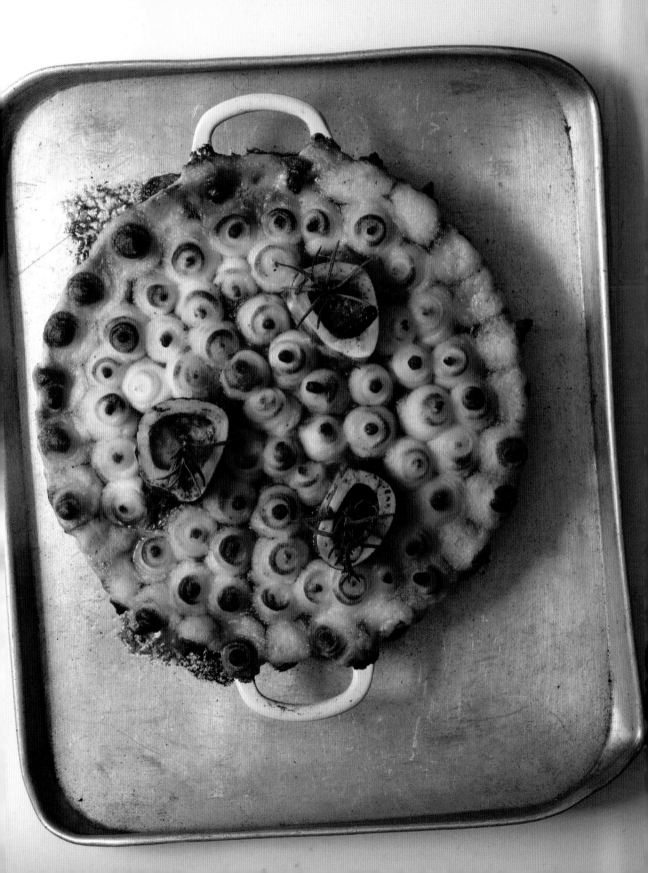

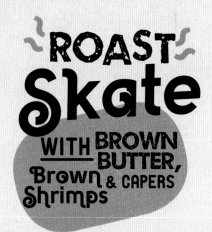

ROAST Skate
WITH BROWN BUTTER, Brown Shrimps & CAPERS

Skate is one special fish and I only eat it every so often, but when I do there's only one way to have it and that's roasted with brown butter and capers. It's a classic and I love it, especially with a few brown shrimps to give the dish a bit of extra texture and sweetness. When it's in season, fine or wild asparagus makes a great addition, too.

70g plain flour, seasoned with
    salt and pepper
2 skate wings, cut into 6
    portions
2 tbsp rapeseed oil
120g butter
150g brown shrimps
60g capers, I prefer vinegared,
    rinsed
150g fine or wild asparagus
    (optional)
juice of 1 lemon
a small handful of parsley,
    finely chopped
sea salt and freshly ground
    black pepper

Preheat the oven to 200°C/Gas 6.

Put the seasoned flour in a bowl. Add the skate and toss in the seasoned flour until evenly coated.

Heat the oil in an ovenproof frying pan with 20g of the butter. When it starts to foam, lay the fish fillets skin-side down in the pan. Add a further 20g of butter and pan-fry the fish for 2–3 minutes on each side, or until crisp and golden. Pop into the oven and finish roasting for 8 minutes. Remove from the pan and place on kitchen paper to drain.

Add the remaining butter to the pan over a medium heat. When it starts to foam, turns a nutty-brown colour and the room fills with an equally nutty aroma, add the brown shrimps, capers and asparagus, if using. Cook for a minute, then add the lemon juice and parsley and season with salt and pepper.

Lay the fish on a plate and cover with a couple of spoonfuls of the burnt butter sauce, brown shrimps, asparagus and capers.

SERVES: 6
PREPARATION TIME: 10 MINUTES
COOKING TIME: 10 MINUTES

WICKED RATING 5

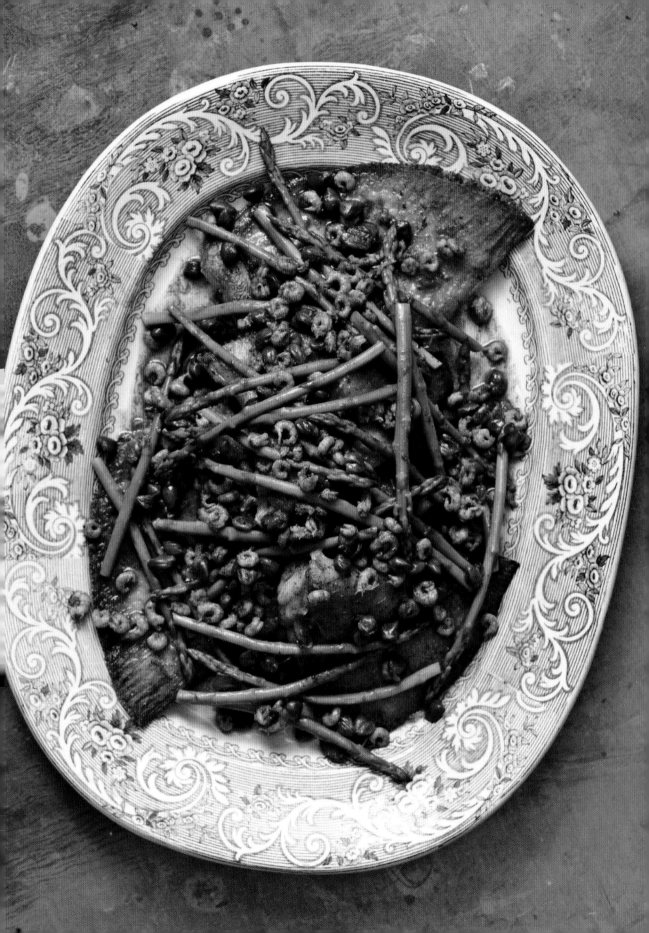

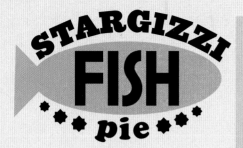

STARGIZZI FISH pie

This is a fish pie to remember! A layer of tarragon pea purée, some delectable little quail eggs and, finally, those star 'Gizzi' prawns help give it the wow factor as well as making it so much tastier than those ordinary versions. It's the perfect Sunday lunch served with a crisp salad of little gem lettuce, chicory, radishes, mint and spring onions.

500g frozen peas
sea salt and freshly ground
    black pepper
1 tbsp finely chopped tarragon,
1 tbsp finely chopped mint
400ml double cream
500g undyed skinless smoked
    haddock fillet
500g skinless pollock fillet
500g skinless salmon fillet
1 ½ litres whole milk
1 bay leaf
5 black peppercorns
1 onion, roughly chopped
12 hard-boiled quail's eggs
1kg potatoes, peeled and cut
    into chunks
20g fresh white breadcrumbs
20g Parmesan, grated
12 raw king prawns, shells
    removed but heads left on

For the sauce
40g butter
40g plain flour
200ml whole milk
50g good-quality cheddar
1 heaped tbsp chopped parsley
1 heaped tbsp chopped dill

Heat the oven to 180°C/Gas 4. Throw the peas into a pan of boiling salted water and cook for 5 minutes. Drain and tip into a blender with the tarragon and mint, 100ml of the cream and a little salt and pepper, then whiz until you get a coarse paté texture. Spread over the base of a 25cm x 20cm ovenproof dish, and leave to cool.

Put the fish fillets in a deep pan, cover with the milk and toss in the bay, peppercorns and onion. Bring the milk just to the boil, then turn off the heat and leave the fish to poach lightly in the milk as it cools. Once cool, strain the fish, reserving the cooking milk. Separate the pieces into large flaky chunks and scatter over the pea purée. Arrange the quail's eggs evenly among the fish.

For the sauce, melt the butter in a pan over a medium heat. Add the flour, stir to form a paste and cook for a minute, then remove from the heat and add 600ml of the reserved fish cooking milk. Beat with a whisk to break down any lumps, then return to the heat and cook, whisking, until the sauce has thickened and is silky smooth. Mix in the cheddar and herbs, then pour over the fish.

Boil the potatoes in a large pan of salted water for 20 minutes. Drain and leave to dry, then mash until really smooth. Add the remaining cream, stir together and season well, then spoon over the fish in an even layer and sprinkle with the breadcrumbs and Parmesan. Push the prawns tail-first into the potato and bake in the oven for 25–30 minutes, until the top is a lovely golden brown and the prawns have turned pink. Serve straight away.

SERVES: 6
PREPARATION
TIME: 40 MINUTES
COOKING TIME:
30 MINUTES

WICKED RATING 8

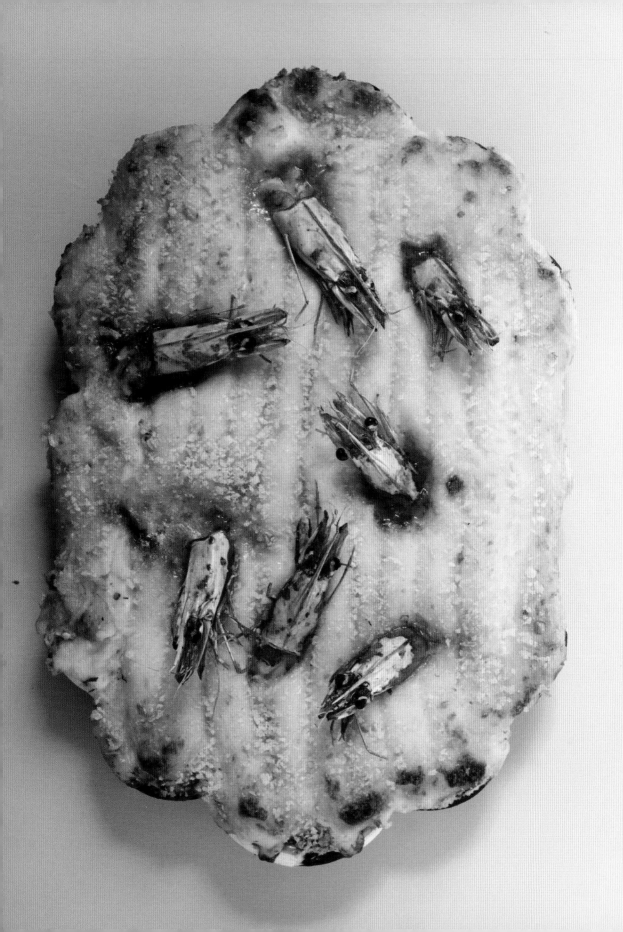

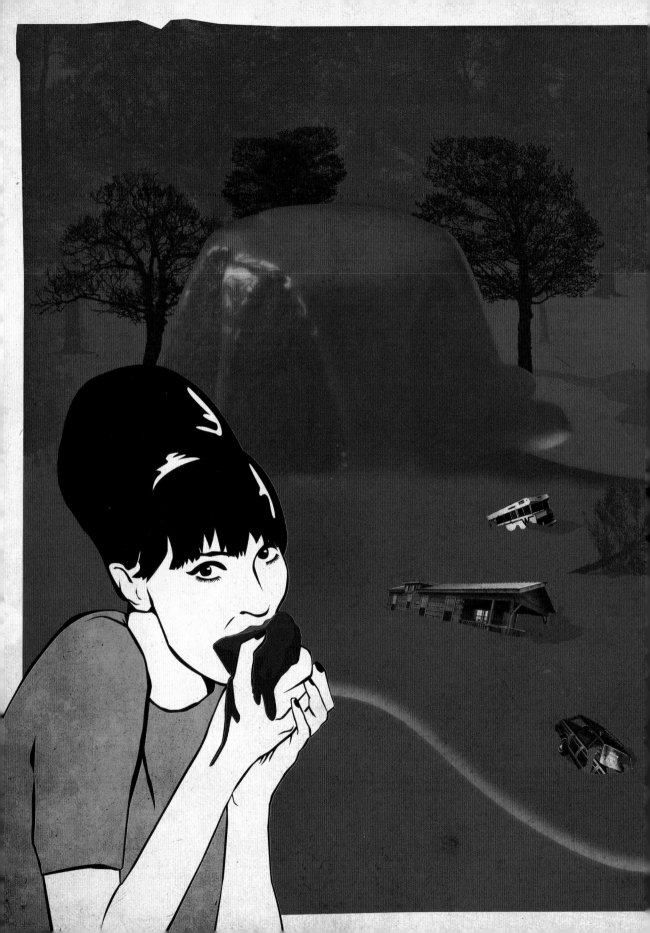

Sweet TREATS

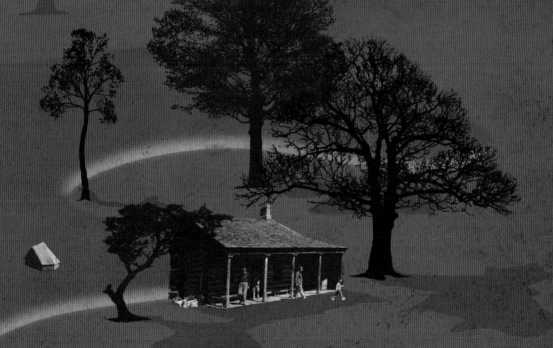

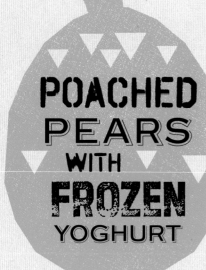

POACHED PEARS WITH FROZEN YOGHURT

When we were growing up, if we were craving a quick dessert, my mum would often reach for a tin of pears. Here I've given this Erskine staple a fancy makeover, poaching fresh pears in a spiced, winey liquour and serving them with my delicious no-fat frozen yoghurt and hot chocolate sauce. To. Die. For. Without the extras the pears weigh in at 160 calories a portion, so would work well as a skinny midweek pud.

For the frozen yoghurt
200g light condensed milk
500g 0% fat Greek yoghurt

For the pears
4 ripe pears (preferably
    Williams or Conference)
zest and juice of 1 orange
200ml Sauternes, or other
    sweet white wine
350ml water
30g runny honey
50g agave nectar
1 vanilla pod, split
4 cardamom pods, bashed
1 tbsp orange-flower water

For the chocolate sauce
100g plain chocolate,
    grated
100ml whole milk
30ml double cream

To make the frozen yoghurt, whisk the condensed milk and Greek yoghurt together. Place the mixture into a pre-chilled ice-cream maker and churn for 45 minutes, or until thickened and starting to solidify. Scrape the mixture into a loaf tin or Tupperware container, pop on the lid or wrap well in clingfilm and freeze overnight until solid. Remove from the freezer about 10–15 minutes before you are ready to serve.

To make the poached pears, peel the pears, leaving the stalk intact, and remove the core from the base using a corer or small melon baller. Cut the orange zest into thin strips. Put all the ingredients in a large saucepan, adding the pears last. Bring to the boil, then reduce the heat to a simmer and cook until the pears are soft, about 5–15 minutes (the time will vary according to the ripeness of the pears). Remove from the heat, transfer the pears and poaching syrup to a bowl and set aside.

To make the chocolate sauce, place the chocolate, milk and cream in a pan and melt gently over a low heat until thick and glossy.

Sit the pears up in bowls and spoon a little of the poaching syrup over each. Pour over the hot chocolate sauce and serve with a scoop or two of frozen yoghurt.

SERVES: 4
PREPARATION TIME: 15 MINUTES
(PLUS OVERNIGHT FREEZING)
COOKING TIME: 15 MINUTES

WICKED RATING 3

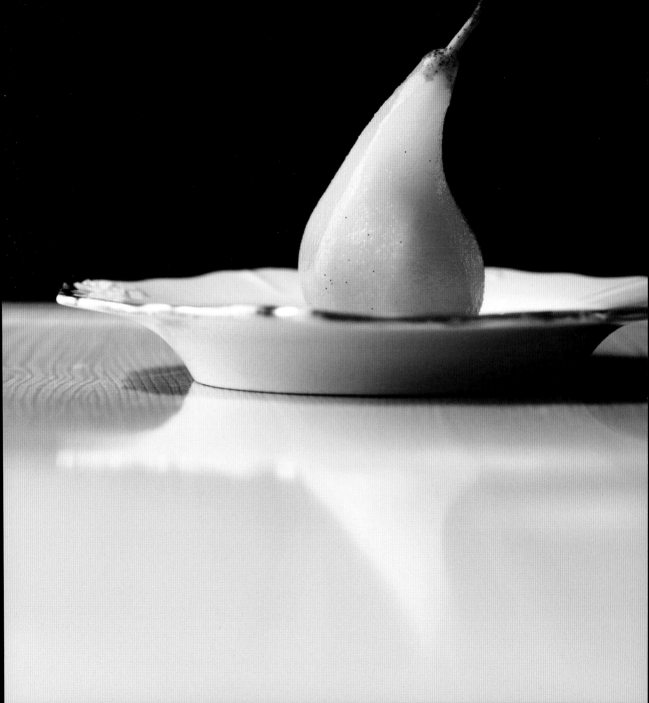

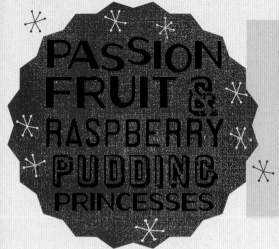

PASSION FRUIT & RASPBERRY PUDDING PRINCESSES

The Queen of Puddings has had a revamp! Served in individual portions, we find the grand old lady reborn with a youthful, light filling of puckering passion fruit curd and fresh raspberries. It's a combination I have won many baking awards with and I've have been told by a number of people that this is the best pudding they have ever eaten. You MUST give it a go.

250ml whole milk
250ml double cream
a few drops of vanilla
    essence
125g golden caster sugar
5 large free-range egg yolks
150g breadcrumbs
zest of 2 lemons
200g fresh raspberries
double cream, to serve

For the passion fruit curd
150ml sieved fresh passion
    fruit juice (from about
    14 passion fruits)
75g golden caster sugar
1 free-range egg, plus 3
    free-range egg yolks
75g unsalted butter

For the meringue
4 large fresh egg whites, at
    room temperature
120g golden caster sugar

Preheat the oven to 160°C/Gas 2.

To make the passion fruit curd, put the juice, sugar and eggs in a bowl set over a pan of simmering water. Stir continuously for 8–10 minutes, or until thickened. Remove from the heat and whisk in the butter. Cover with clingfilm and pop in the fridge to cool and set.

Pour the milk and cream into a pan. Add the vanilla essence and bring slowly to the boil, stirring occasionally. Whisk the sugar and egg yolks together in a large bowl until pale and creamy, then gently pour the egg mix into the hot milk and cream, whisking as you go. Stir in the breadcrumbs and lemon zest.

Pour the pudding mixture into 8 individual ramekins and place these in a roasting tin. Half-fill the tin with hot water (to make a bain marie) and bake for 15–20 minutes, until the batter is just set but with a slight wobble. Remove from the oven and leave to cool. Turn the oven temperature up to 190°C/Gas 5.

While the puds are cooling, make the meringue topping. Whisk the egg whites into stiff peaks, then gradually whisk in the sugar 1 tablespoon at a time, until it is all combined and the mix is firm and glossy.

Split the curd over the top of the puddings and add about 5 raspberries to each. Cover the puddings completely with the meringue mix and shape the tops as you would a cupcake. Bake for 8–10 minutes, until the meringue is golden brown. Serve immediately with double cream.

**SERVES: 8
PREPARATION
TIME: 30 MINUTES
COOKING TIME:
40 MINUTES**

WICKED RATING 5

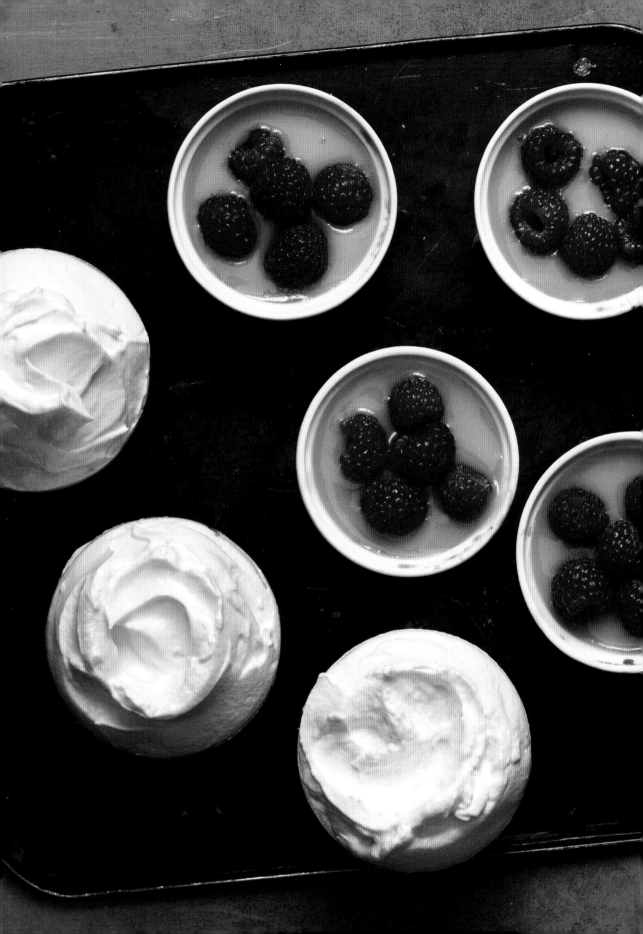

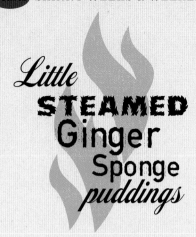

Little STEAMED Ginger Sponge *puddings*

Ginger has to be one of the most traditional flavours in British baking, which is astounding, as we don't grow it here. We can thank the spice trade for this. I like making these scrumptious gingery puds in minis as you get more of the delicious sauce to douse them in. These little beauties won me Pudding Club on a cookery show – I urge you to try them.

150g unsalted butter, at room temperature, plus extra for greasing
130g golden caster sugar
3 free-range eggs
150g self-raising flour
a pinch of salt
$^1/_2$ tsp baking powder
40g fresh white breadcrumbs
3 tbsp milk
2 tbsp chopped stem ginger, plus 2 tbsp of the gingery syrup it comes in
zest and juice of 1 lemon
clotted cream, to serve

For the syrup
25ml King's Ginger Liqueur
juice of 1 lemon
4 tbsp golden syrup
4 tbsp gingery syrup from a jar of stem ginger

Preheat the oven to 200°C/Gas 6.

Cream together the butter and sugar with an electric mixer and whisk until pale and fluffy. Add the eggs one at a time, whisking well between each one, then sift over the flour, salt and baking powder to form a batter. Add the breadcrumbs, milk, ginger, syrup, zest and juice and beat together well. (The mix should be very creamy; add a little more milk to loosen it if you have to.)

Melt together the syrup ingredients in a small pan over a low heat. Grease 8 individual ramekins very well with butter and drop 1 tablespoon of the syrup mixture into the base of each.

Divide the batter between the moulds. Cover each ramekin with a square of pleated buttered foil (the pleat in the middle of the foil will help the foil to expand once the pudding starts to rise) and secure with string.

Place the ramekins in a deep roasting tin half-filled with hot water. Cook in the oven for 30–35 minutes until the puddings have puffed up, are firm to touch and are golden on top. Leave to cool slightly and then turn out. Serve with a big dollop of clotted cream.

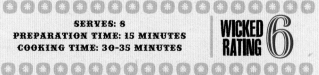

SERVES: 8
PREPARATION TIME: 15 MINUTES
COOKING TIME: 30-35 MINUTES

WICKED RATING 6

BUTTERSCOTCH Delight

I have a soft spot for Angel Delight, that classic, very British, instant custard dessert. I know I'm not alone – every person I speak to about retro puddings from their childhood raves about it. This homemade version tastes just like the packet stuff (though perhaps a bit more grown-up), without any of the things in it that might put you off eating the original!

2 tbsp cornflour
500ml milk
2 free-range eggs,
    separated
110g soft brown sugar
30g unsalted butter
1 tsp vanilla extract

In a large bowl, mix the cornflour with a tablespoon of the milk to make a smooth paste. Bring the remainder of the milk to the boil and pour over the cornflour paste, stirring constantly. Return the mixture to a clean pan and simmer for 2–3 minutes. Remove from the heat and leave for 5 minutes to cool slightly. Mix in the egg yolks and cook without boiling for a further 5 minutes, until the custard mixture leaves a film on the back of a wooden spoon.

Put the sugar in a heavy-based pan and melt over a low heat until it starts to caramelise – you want a nice mahogany-brown colour. Stir in the butter and, once it has melted, add the milk and egg-yolk mix along with the vanilla. Sieve the mixture into a clean bowl to remove any lumps.

In another bowl whisk the egg whites until stiff. Fold 1 large spoonful of the beaten egg white into the sieved custard mixture to loosen it. Gently fold the rest of the egg white into the mixture, being careful not to knock out any air. Spoon into serving dishes and chill for 2 hours before serving.

SERVES: 4
PREPARATION TIME: 10 MINUTES
COOKING TIME: 10 MINUTES
(PLUS 2 HOURS SETTING TIME)

WICKED RATING 4

RICE PUDDING SOUFFLÉ
with STRAWBERRY SAUCE

I first came across this when Tristan Welch showcased it at Taste of London a couple of years ago while I was on the judging panel. It won an award and I was blown away with its deliciousness. I went straight home to work on my variation, which is now a staple in our house. It's a really light way to enjoy rice pudding and the strawberry sauce and cream which fill the middle send its yumminess to stratospheric levels.

500ml full-fat milk
100g pudding rice
1 vanilla pod, cut in
   half lengthways
a good grating of nutmeg
110g caster sugar
unsalted butter,
   for greasing
30g rice flour
the whites of 4 large eggs,
   about 125g, at room
   temperature
100ml pouring cream,
   to serve

For the sauce
100g fresh strawberries
2 tbsp icing sugar

To make the sauce, put the berries and sugar in a blender and blitz until smooth. Pass through a sieve to remove any bits, transfer to a serving jug and set aside until needed.

Heat the milk, rice, vanilla pod and nutmeg in a small saucepan and slowly bring to the boil. Turn down the temperature and cook over a low heat for 30 minutes. Add 80g of the sugar and continue to cook for another 10 minutes, or until the rice is soft and the mixture has thickened and become gooey. Leave to cool completely.

Preheat the oven to 190°C/Gas 5. Grease four large or six small ramekins with butter. Combine the remaining caster sugar, a little extra nutmeg and the rice flour and use to dust the ramekins.

Pour the rice pudding into a clean metal bowl. In a separate bowl, whisk the egg whites to medium peaks. Using a large metal spoon, fold one-third of the beaten egg mix into the rice pudding to lighten it, then gently fold in the remainder.

Spoon the soufflé mixture up to the brim of your prepared ramekins and bake until risen and golden brown on top, about 8–10 minutes for smaller ones and 12–14 minutes for larger ones. Serve immediately, poking a hole in the centre of each soufflé and pouring in the strawberry sauce and cream at the table.

SERVES: 4-6
PREPARATION
TIME: 10 MINUTES
COOKING TIME:
1 HOUR

WICKED RATING 6

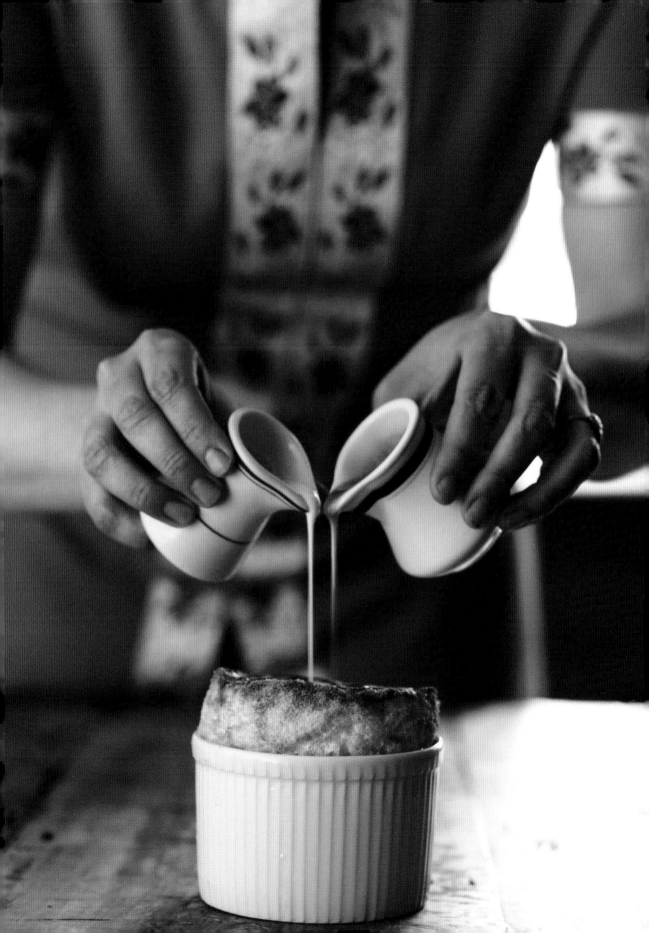

RHUBARB & PIMM'S TRIFLE

The two things that I get cravings for in early spring are rhubarb and Pimm's. It must be something to do with the sun coming through the window... Rhubarb and Pimm's are brilliant together, rhubarb and ginger (cake) are a marriage made in heaven and rhubarb and custard are practically family – you just know this is going to be a goody.

50ml Pimm's
50ml dry sherry
50g caster sugar
1 x 600ml pot of fresh custard
300ml double cream
1 tsp icing sugar
50g good-quality dark chocolate
a few glacé cherries (if you fancy)

For the ginger cake
225g butter, plus extra for greasing
225g dark brown sugar
225g black treacle
2 eggs, beaten
290ml milk
340g plain flour
1 tbsp ground ginger
1 tbsp ground cinnamon
a small grating of nutmeg
2 tsp bicarbonate of soda

For the rhubarb jelly
500g rhubarb, trimmed and cut into 3cm chunks
150ml water
140g caster sugar
50ml Pimm's
4 gelatine leaves

To make the ginger cake, preheat the oven to 160°C/Gas 2. Grease and line a 30cm x 20cm roasting tin. Melt the butter, sugar and treacle together in a pan, leave to cool for 10 minutes, then stir in the eggs and milk. Sift the flour, ginger, cinnamon, nutmeg and bicarbonate of soda together in a large mixing bowl, then fold in the butter mixture to form a batter. Pour the batter into the roasting tin and bake in the oven for 45 minutes, or until the cake is risen and firm. Leave to cool on a wire rack and store in an airtight container until needed.

To make the jelly, preheat the oven to 200°C/Gas 6. Put the rhubarb in an ovenproof dish. Add the water, sugar and Pimm's and cook in the oven for 15 minutes, or until the rhubarb is just tender. Strain the rhubarb juice into a small saucepan. Soak the gelatine leaves in cold water for 10 minutes, squeeze out any water with your hands and stir into the rhubarb juice to dissolve. Put the rhubarb in your trifle bowl, pour over the liquid and refrigerate for at least 4 hours to set.

Now you're ready to put the trifle together. Combine the Pimm's, Sherry and caster sugar. Chop up 150g of the cake into cubes, add it to the boozy mix and then pop on top of the rhubarb jelly. Pour over the custard and level out the top. Whisk the cream together with the icing sugar until it is gently holding its shape, then use to top the custard. Grate over the chocolate and finish with glacé cherries if you like. Pop in the fridge to chill for 1 hour before eating.

SERVES: 6
PREPARATION TIME: 30 MINUTES
COOKING TIME: 1 HOUR
(PLUS 5 HOURS SETTING/CHILLING TIME)

WICKED RATING 7

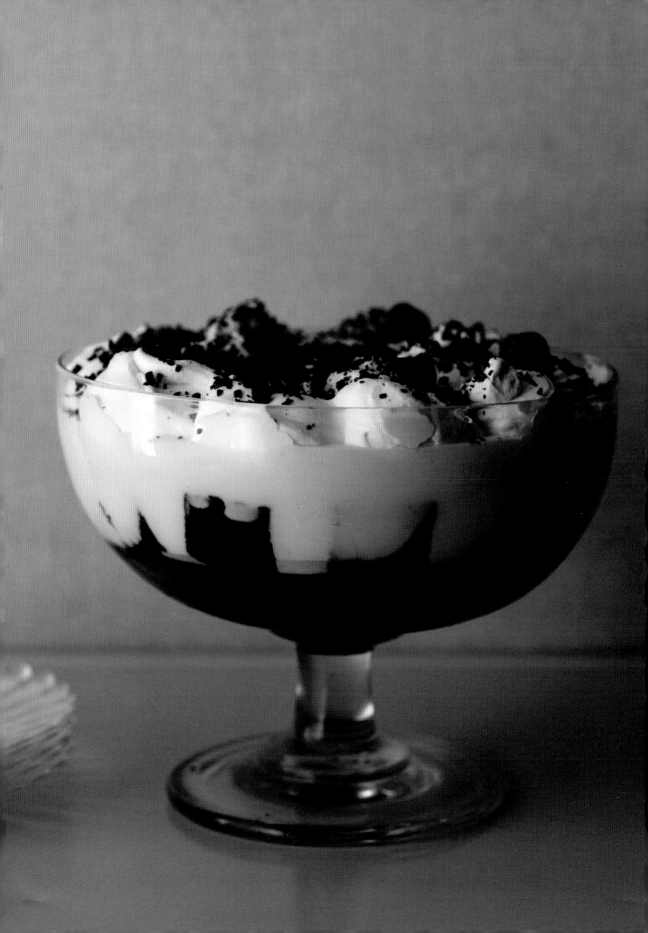

CÀ PHÊ DÁ
Cheesecake

Cà phê dá is a Vietnamese iced coffee, but one made with condensed milk rather than the ordinary stuff. Superbly creamy but with a delicious toffee backbone, it tastes a million bucks – and happens to make for a rather lovely cheesecake too...

For the base
85ml melted butter, plus
    extra for greasing
200g digestive biscuits,
    whizzed to fine crumbs
    in a food processor
1 tbsp golden caster sugar

For the filling
3 x 300g tubs full-fat cream
    cheese
1 x 400g can condensed
    milk
50g muscovado sugar
3 tbsp plain flour
1 tsp vanilla extract
5–6 tbsp extra-strong
    espresso coffee
2–3 tbsp Kahlúa
3 large free-range eggs,
    plus 1 egg yolk

Preheat the oven to 160ºC/Gas 2. Line the base of a 23cm springform cake tin with baking paper and grease the sides.

For the biscuit base, stir the melted butter into the biscuit crumbs and sugar until evenly mixed. Press the mixture into the base of the tin and bake for 10 minutes. Leave to cool while you prepare the filling.

Raise the oven temperature to 200ºC/Gas 6. In a food processor, beat the cream cheese until smooth, then gradually add the condensed milk, sugar, flour, vanilla extract, coffee and Kahlúa. Whisk in the eggs and yolk, one at a time. The filling should be smooth, light and a little airy.

Pour the filling into the tin and bake for 20 minutes, then reduce the oven temperature to 100ºC/Gas ½ and bake for a further 25 minutes, or until the filling wobbles slightly when you gently shake the tin. When it has reached this point, turn off the oven and open the door for a cheesecake that's creamy in the centre, or leave it closed if you prefer a drier texture. Either way, leave it to cool in the oven for 2 hours. The cheesecake may crack slightly on top as it cools.

Once cool, cover the cheesecake loosely with foil and refrigerate for at least 8 hours or overnight. When ready to serve, run a round-bladed knife around the inside of the tin to loosen any stuck edges. Unlock the side of the tin and slide the cheesecake off the bottom onto a plate, slipping the baking paper out from underneath before serving.

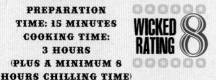

SERVES: 12
PREPARATION
TIME: 15 MINUTES
COOKING TIME:
3 HOURS
(PLUS A MINIMUM 8
HOURS CHILLING TIME)

WICKED
RATING 8

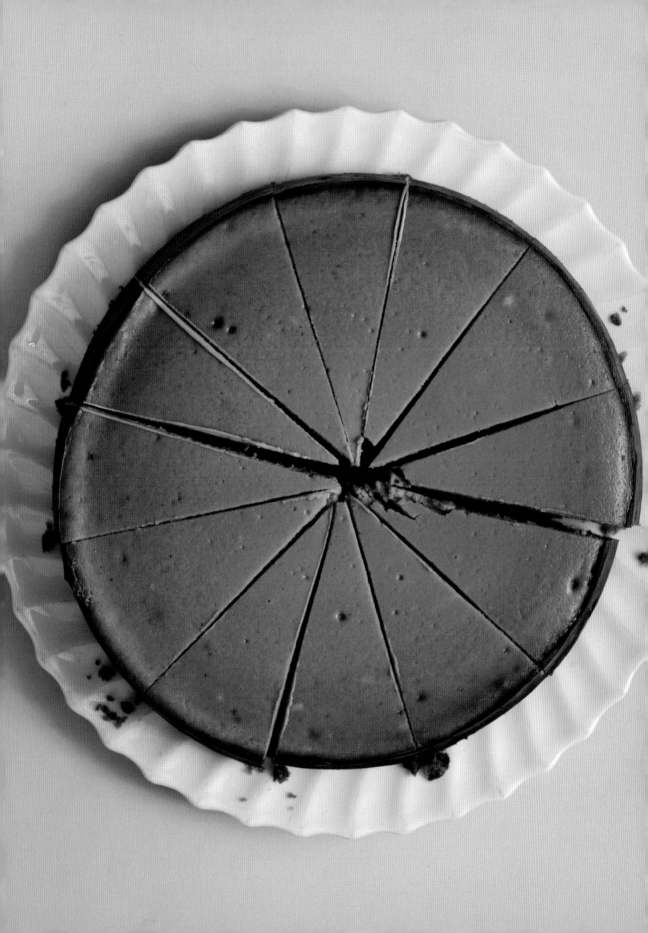

Gypsy TART

1 x 410g tin evaporated
    milk, refrigerated
    overnight
275g light muscovado sugar
a good pinch of vanilla salt
    (optional)
crème fraîche and fresh
    berries, to serve

For the pastry:
225g plain flour
a pinch of salt
150g cold butter, chopped,
    plus extra for greasing
1 medium egg, beaten
25ml cold water

Like pretty much everyone from Kent, if you ask my other half what food reminds him most of his childhood he'll say gypsy tart. Some of us may know it as the caramel slice we used to get at school – think thin pastry covered in a slick of toffee with the best sticky skin. I have seen and tried making this recipe as a thick tart but it doesn't work, so I've gone back to doing it as a tray bake, like I used to have at school. There's something delightfully retro about it, though I do serve it the modern way with the sharpness of crème fraîche and fresh berries to cut through the tart's sweetness.

To make the pastry, sift the flour and salt into a bowl. Add the butter and rub in with your fingers until the mixture resembles breadcrumbs. (If you'd rather save time, you can whiz these together in a food processor instead). Add the egg and water and mix into a smooth dough. Cover in clingfilm and leave to rest in the fridge for at least 30 minutes.

Preheat the oven to 200°C/Gas 6. Roll out the pastry and use it to line a 40cm x 20cm rectangular baking tray, drawing the pastry up at the sides to make a shallow tart case. Line the pastry with greaseproof paper, fill with ceramic baking beans and bake blind for 15–20 minutes. Remove the beans and paper and leave the pastry in the tray to cool. Reduce the oven temperature to 180°C/Gas 4.

Using an electric mixer, whisk together the chilled evaporated milk, sugar and vanilla salt, if using, for 12–15 minutes, until the mix resembles softly whipped, coffee-coloured cream. Pour it into the pastry case and bake for 10 minutes, until the filling has set and the surface is sticky. Remove from the oven and leave to cool to room temperature. Slice into rectangles and serve with crème fraîche and fresh berries.

SERVES: 6
PREPARATION
TIME: 25 MINUTES
COOKING TIME:
45 MINUTES

WICKED RATING 9

POLISH *Damson* DOUGHNUTS

110g caster sugar
330ml warm milk
30g melted butter
30g lemon juice
30g dark rum
1 free-range egg yolk
1 tsp salt
200g plain flour
350g white bread flour
1 x 7g sachet fast-action
    yeast
vegetable oil, for oiling
    and deep frying
1 x 370g jar prune or
    damson jam, sieved to
    remove lumps

My grandfather was Polish and, though my Mum doesn't speak the language or hasn't ever been, we were always given our fill of Polish food growing up. I particularly loved the pastries, with the **pounchki** – the prune (or sometimes damson) doughnuts – being my favourite. As everyone seems to have a different recipe for them, I tested a whole bunch to come up with these guys. They are really easy to make and are a great way of using up a seasonal jam.

Put 60g of the sugar into a big bowl with all the rest of the ingredients except for the vegetable oil and jam. Mix together well to form a dough, then transfer to a floured surface and knead for 5 minutes, until the dough is soft and flexible. Place into an oiled mixing bowl and cover with clingfilm. Leave it in a warm place, such as an airing cupboard or near a warm cooker, for 1–2 hours, until doubled in size.

Remove the clingfilm and, using your fist, knock all the air out of the inflated dough. Divide and roll the dough into golf-ball-sized pieces, then place them on a lined baking sheet, leaving a good 3cm space between each. Cover with an oiled sheet of clingfilm and leave for 30–45 minutes, until trebled in size.

Fill your deep-fat fryer or large saucepan with vegetable oil (if using a pan, only fill to two-thirds of the way up the side). In batches of about 5 at a time, lower the doughnuts into the oil, and deep-fry for 3–4 minutes, turning them halfway through cooking, until golden brown. Remove with a slotted spoon and place on kitchen paper.

Toss the doughnuts in the remaining sugar, making sure they get completely covered. Load the jam into a piping bag fitted with a small plain tip and use to fill the doughnuts. Serve warm.

**MAKES: 15 DOUGHNUTS
PREPARATION TIME: 20 MINUTES (PLUS 1-2 HOURS RISING TIME)
COOKING TIME: 10 MINUTES**

WICKED RATING 8

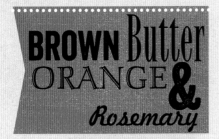

BROWN Butter ORANGE & Rosemary

CHOCOLATE CHIP Cookies

In my last book, I think the recipe that came up trumps was my millionaire's shortbread with rosemary-infused salted caramel, and here we are on a similar theme. However weird it sounds, the rosemary, orange and chocolate combine fantastically, while the brown butter adds a delicious nuttiness to these decidedly grown-up cookies.

170g unsalted butter
180g muscovado sugar
100g golden caster sugar
the zest of 1–2 oranges
3 sprigs of rosemary, leaves removed and very finely chopped
1 egg, plus 1 egg yolk
225g plain flour
½ tsp baking powder
¼ tsp bicarbonate of soda
½ tsp salt
300g good-quality milk chocolate, cut into bite-sized chunks

Gently heat the butter in a saucepan. until nutty brown. At this point, whip it off the heat, pour it into a mixing bowl and leave to cool for 15 minutes.

Whisk the cooled butter together with the sugars, orange zest and rosemary for 2–3 minutes, or until the mixture is light and fluffy. Add in the egg and yolk and beat for a further 7–8 minutes, then add the flour, baking powder, bicarbonate of soda and salt and gently mix together to form a dough. Add the chocolate chunks and mix until just incorporated.

Portion out the dough into small walnut-sized pieces onto a lined baking tray, ensuring there is a 4cm radius space between dough pieces. Pat the dough flat, wrap the tray tightly in clingfilm and refrigerate for an hour.

Preheat the oven to 180°C/Gas 4. Bake the cookies for 10–12 minutes, until very faintly browned on the edges but still bright yellow in the centre. Cool the cookies completely on the baking tray before transferring to a plate or an airtight container for storage until needed.

MAKES: 12 COOKIES
PREPARATION TIME: 15 MINUTES
(PLUS 1 HOUR CHILLING TIME)
COOKING TIME: 10–12 MINUTES

WICKED RATING 7

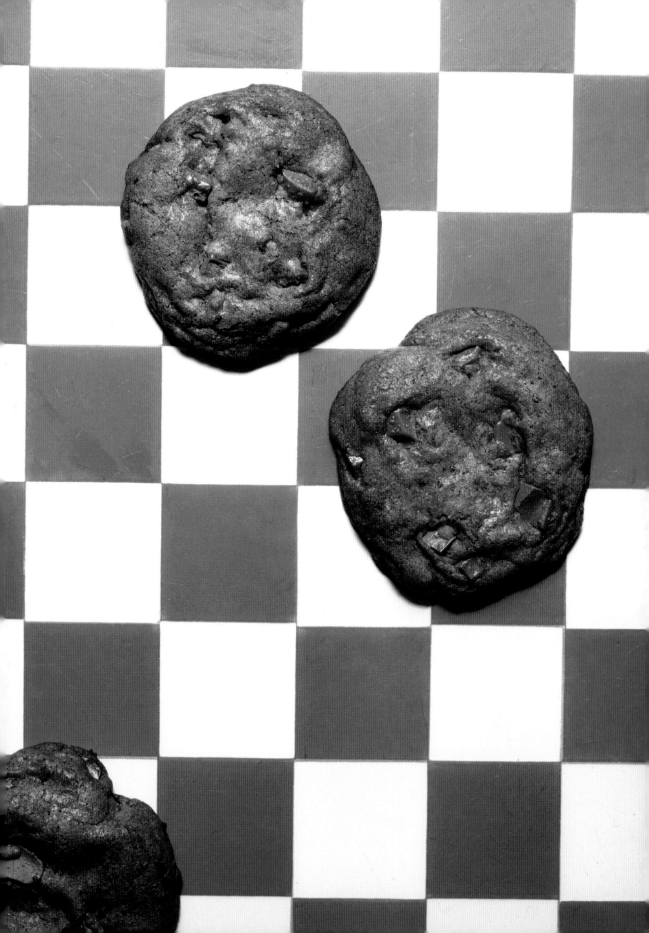

PASSION FRUIT BLUEBERRY AND Poppy Seed MUFFINS

The flavour of passion fruit is without doubt one of my favourites, though needless to say if you don't want to make the curd you could use a good shop-bought lemon, lime or orange one in its place.

225g self-raising flour
50g muesli or oats
75g golden caster sugar
1 tsp baking powder
¼ tsp bicarbonate of soda
a pinch of sea salt
2 tbsp poppy seeds
zest of 2 lemons
200ml milk
75ml lemon juice
125g unsalted butter,
    melted
1 free-range egg
250g passion fruit curd
    (p170)
150g blueberries

Preheat the oven to 180ºC/Gas 4.

Mix the flour, muesli or oats, sugar, baking powder, bicarbonate of soda, salt, poppy seeds and lemon zest together in a large bowl.

In a separate bowl, mix the milk and lemon juice together. Give it a good stir – within a few seconds you will see it start to separate and the milk thicken. Add the butter, egg and 100g of the passion fruit curd and give it a quick mix. Pour into the flour mix and stir until combined, then add the blueberries.

Load a muffin tray with 8 tulip muffin cases. Divide the mixture among the cases (an ice-cream scoop comes in handy for this if you have one).

Load the remaining passion fruit curd into a piping bag. Pipe about 2 teapoons of curd into the centre of each muffin mix, adding a little splodge on top as you draw the nozzle out of each.

Pop the muffins in the oven and bake for 25–30 minutes until they have puffed up and gone golden and the curd has sunk a little (they'll look a little like those amazing Portuguese custard tarts). Remove from the oven and leave to cool before serving.

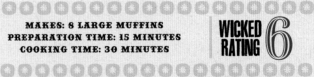

MAKES: 8 LARGE MUFFINS
PREPARATION TIME: 15 MINUTES
COOKING TIME: 30 MINUTES

WICKED RATING 6

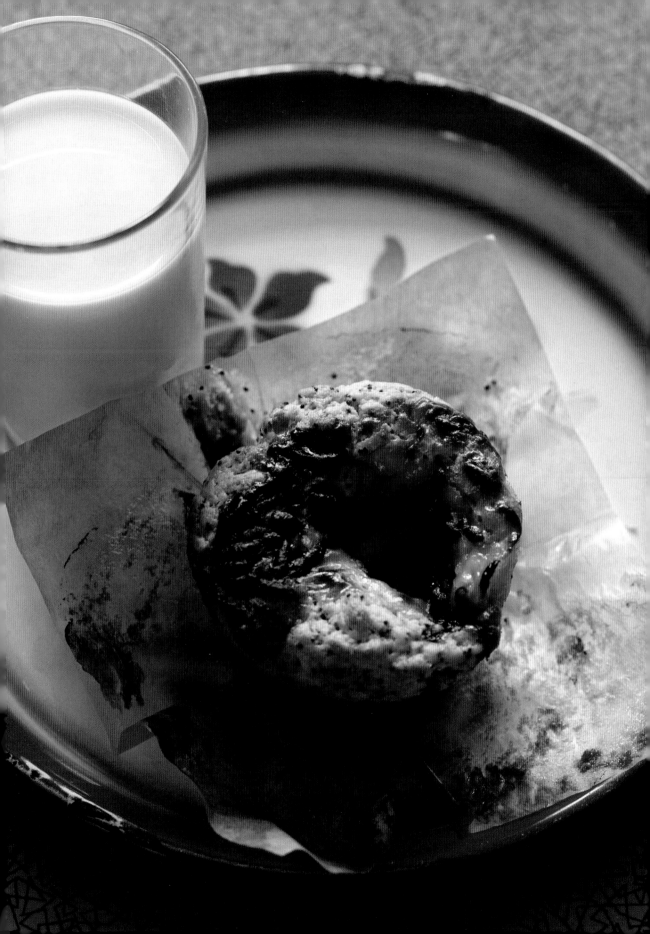

SPICED PUMPKIN CAKE with VANILLA CREAM CHEESE FROSTING

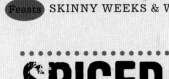

Last time I touched down in NYC I hit the Magnolia Bakery. It was Thanksgiving and they were overflowing with spiced pumpkin cupcakes. Adding pumpkin to sweet food is the norm in the States and it really gives a boost of sweetness and moisture, meaning you don't need to add so much sugar or fat. Bingo! Think carrot cake but with a bit more va va voom.

butter, for greasing
100g light brown
    muscovado sugar
50ml rapeseed oil
1 tsp vanilla extract
1 free-range egg
110g plain flour
½ tsp cinnamon
a pinch of allspice
a good pinch of ground
    ginger
¼ tsp bicarbonate of soda
¼ tsp baking powder
25g chopped walnuts
100g fresh pumpkin or
    butternut squash,
    peeled, deseeded and
    grated
1 tbsp milk

For the cream cheese
    frosting
100g cream cheese
50g icing sugar
½ tsp vanilla extract
50ml double cream
50g plain chocolate, grated

Heat the oven to 170°C/Gas 3. Grease and line a 15cm round cake tin.

Put the sugar, oil and vanilla into a large bowl and beat with an electric whisk for 2 minutes to combine. Add the egg and whisk for another 2 minutes.

In a separate bowl, sift together the flour, cinnamon, allspice, ginger, bicarbonate of soda and baking powder. Add the walnuts and, using a large metal spoon, fold the dry mixture into the wet until just combined. This will result in a very thick batter.

Fold the pumpkin and milk into the batter, spoon it into the tin and bake for 30 minutes. The cake is ready when it is golden and a toothpick inserted into it comes out clean. Leave to cool in the tin for 10 minutes, then transfer it to a wire rack to cool completely.

To make the frosting, lightly whip the cream cheese until smooth. Sift over the icing sugar, add the vanilla extract and beat together. Separately whip the cream until it just begins to thicken but still holds it shape. Add the cream to the cream-cheese mix and beat again until combined. Top the cake with the frosting and sprinkle over the grated chocolate to finish.

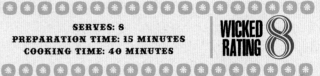

SERVES: 8
PREPARATION TIME: 15 MINUTES
COOKING TIME: 40 MINUTES

WICKED RATING 8

HENI'S PEAR & GINGER CAKE

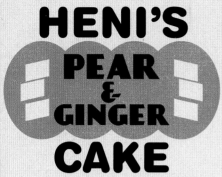

My sister Heni loves to bake. My sister Heni loves ginger and pears. So it made perfect sense to name this rich and sticky dark ginger cake, stuffed full of boozy dried pears, after her. I've made the frosting optional as the cake doesn't actually need it, but if you want to make it that bit more opulent, then go forth and frost!

8 dried pears
3–5 tbsp King's Ginger Liqueur, Poire William or Cointreau
zest and juice of 1 orange
zest and juice of 1 lemon
125g self-raising flour
½ tsp bicarbonate of soda
½ tbsp ground ginger
½ tsp cinnamon
¼ tsp mixed spice
a grating of nutmeg
75g butter
50g black treacle
75g golden syrup
75g light muscovado sugar
1 tbsp milk
1 free-range egg
2 tbsp stem ginger, finely chopped, plus 2 tbsp of the syrup it comes in and extra for garnish (optional)

For the frosting (optional)
100g cream cheese
50g icing sugar
zest of 1 orange
50ml double cream

Put the dried pears in a bowl with the booze, zest and juices and leave overnight to soak.

Heat the oven to 180°C/Gas 4. Line a 15cm round cake tin with greaseproof paper. Mix together the flour, bicarbonate of soda and spices in a bowl.

Melt the butter in a pan, add the treacle, golden syrup, sugar and milk and mix together well. Stir the treacle mixture into the dry mix along with the egg and stem ginger.

Remove the soaked pears from the booze and chop roughly. Fold the chopped pear into the cake mix along with 2 tablespoons of the alcohol, scooping up and adding as much of the zest as you can.

Carefully pour the cake mixture into the tin, pushing the pears right into the mixture. Bake for 1 hour. The cake is ready when you can slide a skewer into it and it comes out clean. Remove the cake from the oven and leave to cool in the tin for 15 minutes, then transfer it to a wire rack to cool completely.

If you're going to make the frosting, lightly whip the cream cheese until smooth. Sieve over the icing sugar, add the orange zest and beat together. Whip the cream in a separate bowl until it just begins to thicken but still holds its shape, then add to the cream cheese mix and beat again until combined. Top the cake with the frosting, then sprinkle over a little more chopped ginger.

SERVES: 8
PREPARATION TIME: 15 MINUTES (PLUS 24 HOURS SOAKING TIME)
COOKING TIME: 1 HOUR

WICKED RATING 8

•ELYSE'S• PEANUT BUTTER & CORNFLAKE BROWNIES

By now I'm sure you've grasped how I'm totally inspired by American food in all its bonkersness, so when I met the exceptionally talented Elyse of Lallapolosa Bakery and she introduced me to her peanut butter and cornflake brownies, I blew my top! These brownies are off-the-Richter-scale wicked – but if you need that sugar splurge, why not do it in style?

250g unsalted butter
150g good-quality dark chocolate, chopped into small pieces
200g golden caster sugar
100g best-quality cocoa powder
2 tsp instant espresso granules
70g plain flour
1 tsp salt
1 tbsp vanilla extract
4 large free-range eggs, beaten

For the peanut butter layer
340g chunky peanut butter
250g unsalted butter
200g light muscovado sugar
1 tsp salt
1 tsp vanilla extract
150g icing sugar
150g cornflakes

For the topping
200g milk or plain chocolate
30g butter

Preheat the oven to 180°C/Gas 4.

To make the peanut butter layer, put the peanut butter, butter, muscovado sugar, salt and vanilla extract in a pan and heat until completely melted and just beginning to bubble, stirring constantly. Make sure you watch it as it burns super quick! Remove from the heat and add the icing sugar a little at a time, stirring, until completely combined. Stir in the cornflakes, then pop in a blender and pulse until the mix starts to break up but still has crispy shards of cornflake running through. Set aside.

To make the brownies, melt the butter and dark chocolate chunks together in a bowl over a small pan of gently simmering water (aka a bain marie). Put the sugar, cocoa powder, espresso granules, flour, salt and vanilla in a separate bowl and mix until well combined. Stir in the eggs, then add the melted chocolate and mix together with 4 or 5 swift swoops. Pour into a 30cm x 20cm greased and lined brownie tin and bake in the oven for 20 minutes, or until it cracks across the top but the brownies should still be slightly gooey in the middle. When the cake is cool enough to touch, spread over the peanut butter layer neatly. Leave to cool.

For the chocolate topping, melt the chocolate and butter together in a bain marie as before. Pour over the cooled peanut butter layer, smooth out and pop it in the fridge to set. Cut into squares and store in an airtight container.

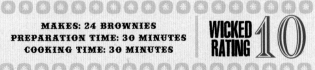

MAKES: 24 BROWNIES
PREPARATION TIME: 30 MINUTES
COOKING TIME: 30 MINUTES

WICKED RATING 10

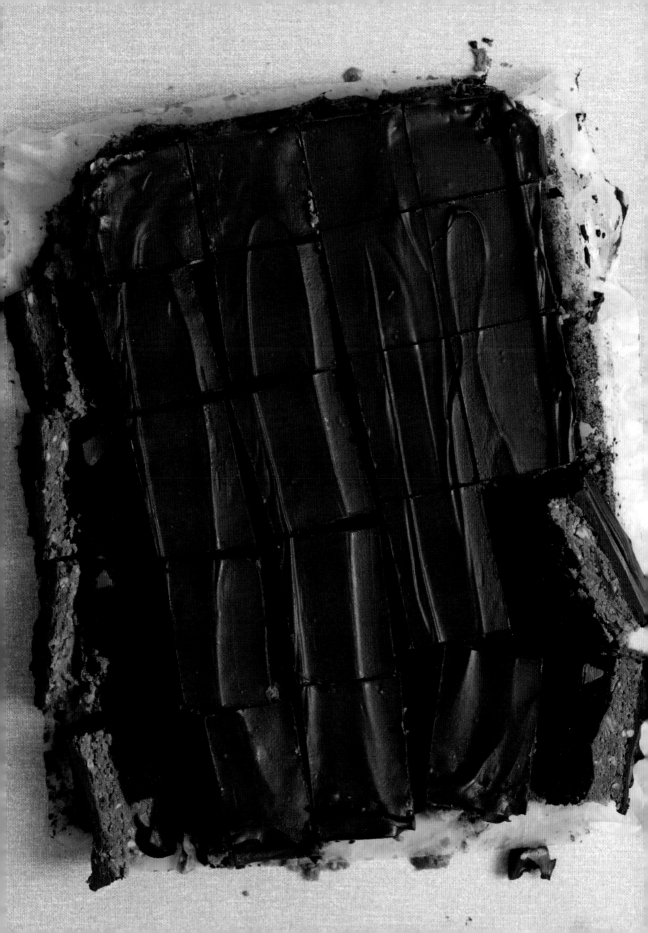

index

acknowledgements

Normally when I write acknowledgments I start with my family, my crutch when writing any of my books, but this time I have to jump straight in and thank the team at Quadrille. Firstly I would like to thank Alison Cathie and Jane O'Shea for commissioning Skinny Weeks & Weekend Feasts. It was a strong idea but your help in fine-tuning it has been invaluable.

This book was written during the craziest busy time of my life. SO I must thank the whole team for their patience with me in the delivery of the book a couple of months, (okay half a year) late. I need to thank you all for dealing with my strong mind. I have big ideas, and as you all know I find it hard to articulate them sometimes. Simon Davis, you have been like my right arm over the last few months – the only person other than my boyfriend and mother who I speak to about a hundred times a day. You have helped me shift and shape the book and make sense of all of my thoughts.

Helen Lewis, David Eldridge and Dean Martin for bringing the book to life. B-movie is not the most conventional brief for a cookbook, but I am thrilled with the results and I think we've managed to make it look like nothing else out there. I hope you feel like it was worth all the to-ing and fro-ing and that we have a beautiful book.

A huge thank you to Jason Lowe (J-Lowe) for your beautiful photographs. You are a master at what you do and I learned so much from you. Thank you for your honesty and guidance and also thank you for the endless cups of THE BEST coffee and lunches from the Towpath Cafe!

Louisa Carter, you were a saving grace. A terrific food stylist, organized in a way I can only dream of and with a superb eye for detail. I loved our chats and thank you for instilling me with confidence. In the same note Cynthia Inions, for prop styling the book. You are like a magpie drawn towards stunning things. You nailed it and I just love being around you.

Fiona Hunter, we've been buddies for a while and you know I think you're the best nutritionalist on the block as we've been working together for yonks, but I feel like having you reaffirm my message in this book makes it all the stronger. Thank you.

I must thank my fellow cooks and friends Stevie Parle, Adam Byatt, Tristan Welsh, Sabrina Ghayour, Reiko Hashimoto, Elyse from Lallopolosa bakery for their delicious recipes and contributions to the book. Your food has been an inspiration to me, which is why I wanted to spread the word!

To team Gizzi; Severine Berman, Tim Beaumont, Jonathan Shalit, Nazli, Dolaps, Sami Knight and Lily Keys. Thank you for taking the best possible care of me. Sev and Tim, you are not only the people who manage me but two of my best friends. I love you both with everything I have.

Now my family. Dean again, this one was a toughy as it was the first time you have had to work with me and my crazy work brain, so not only did you have to live with a crazed nutter you had to work with her too. I don't know if it's possible to cherish something in the way I cherish you. I wake up everyday, look at you, and pinch myself that you're my boyfriend. To my mother Maria; I bore the pants of everyone I meet by constantly banging on about you being my inspiration, but it's true – you are, not just because your food is incredible but growing up you showed me how to be an independent strong woman. Heni and Cora, my sisters, who constantly remind me to never get above my station – you two are my everything. To Edie and Sholto for being the guys who kept me sane and not giving a shit that I'm on telly, just that you're happiest with me showing you how to make biscuits or crawl on the floor pretending to be a monster. To Matt, Keiron, Bingo, Gove, Kate, James, JD, Carl, Glynn and Martha for simply constantly supporting me in everything I do in friendship and food.